SELF-ASSESSMENT IN OBSTETRICS AND GYNAECOLOGY

by Ten Teachers

On the Medical Students reading list 2016

SELF ASSESSMENT IN OBSTETRICS AND GYNAECOLOGY

by Ten Teachers

EMQs, MCQs, SBAs, SAQs and OSCEs

2nd edition

Catherine E. M. Aiken MB/BChir MA PhD MRCP
Academic Clinical Fellow, Department of Obstetrics and Gynaecology, The Rosie Maternity Hospital, Addenbrooke's University Hospital NHS Trust, Cambridge, UK

Jeremy C. Brockelsby MRCOG PhD
Consultant in Obstetrics and Fetal-Maternal Medicine, The Rosie Maternity Hospital, Addenbrooke's University Hospital NHS Trust, Cambridge, UK

Christian Phillips DM MRCOG
Consultant Obstetrician and Gynaecologist and Clinical Director, Maternity and Gynaecology, The North Hampshire Hospital, Basingstoke and North Hampshire NHS Foundation Trust, Basingstoke, UK

Louise C. Kenny MRCOG PhD
Professor of Obstetrics and Consultant Obstetrician and Gynaecologist, The Anu Research Centre, Cork University Maternity Hospital, Department of Obstetrics and Gynaecology, University College Cork, Cork, Ireland

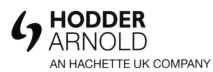

HODDER ARNOLD
AN HACHETTE UK COMPANY

First published in Great Britain in 2007

This second edition published in Great Britain in 2012 by
Hodder Arnold, an imprint of Hodder Education, a division of Hachette UK
338 Euston Road, London NW1 3BH

http://www.hoddereducation.com

Hachette UK's policy is to use papers that are natural, renewable and recyclable products and made from wood grown in sustainable forests. The logging and manufacturing processes are expected to conform to the environmental regulations of the country of origin.

Whilst the advice and information in this book are believed to be true and accurate at the date of going to press, neither the author[s] nor the publisher can accept any legal responsibility or liability for any errors or omissions that may be made. In particular (but without limiting the generality of the preceding disclaimer) every effort has been made to check drug dosages; however it is still possible that errors have been missed. Furthermore, dosage schedules are constantly being revised and new side effects recognized. For these reasons the reader is strongly urged to consult the drug companies' printed instructions before administering any of the drugs recommended in this book.

British Library Cataloguing in Publication Data
A catalogue record for this book is available from the British Library

Library of Congress Cataloging-in-Publication Data
A catalog record for this book is available from the Library of Congress

ISBN-13   978-1-444-17051-1

1 2 3 4 5 6 7 8 9 10

Commissioning Editor:	Joanna Koster
Project Editor:	Joanna Silman
Production Controller:	Francesca Wardell
Cover Design:	Amina Dudhia
Indexer:	Dr. Laurence Errington

Typeset in Minion Regular 9.5 pts by Datapage (India) Pvt. Ltd.
Printed and bound by CPI Group (UK) Ltd., Croydon, CRO 4YY.

Contents

Acknowledgements

The Editor (LCK) would like to acknowledge the help of Mr Fred English, BSc (Hons) with the preparation of this text.

This book is dedicated to my sons, Conor and Eamon (LCK)
To my Father and to Oscar (CA)

Commonly used abbreviations

ABO	ABO blood group
AC	abdominal circumference
ACTH	adrenocorticotrophin horome
ADH	antidiuretic hormone
AFP	alpha-fetoprotein
AIDS	acquired immunodeficiency syndrome
ALT	alanine aminotransferase
AMH	anti-Müllerian hormone
AP	anterior–posterior
BMI	body mass index
BP	blood pressure
BPD	biparietal diameter
BSO	bilateral salpingo-oophorectomy
BV	bacterial vaginosis
CAH	congenital adrenal hyperplasia
CGIN	cervical glandular intraepithelial neoplasia
CIN	cervical intraepithelial neoplasia
CMV	congenital cytomegalovirus
COCP	combined oral contraceptive pill
CPD	cephalopelvic disproportion
CT	computed tomography
CTG	cardiotocography
CVS	chorionic villus sampling
DFA	direct fluorescent antibody
DVT	deep vein thrombosis
ECG	electrocardiogram
ECV	external cephalic version
EDD	expected date of delivery
ELISA	enzyme-linked immunosorbent assay
FBC	full blood count
FL	femur length
FSH	follicle-stimulating hormone
FTA	fluorescent treponemal antibody
GFR	glomerular filtration rate
GnRH	gonadotrophin-releasing hormone
GP	general practitioner
HbF	haemoglobin F
HC	head circumference
HCG	human chorionic gonadotrophin
HDL	high-density lipoprotein
HELLP	haemolysis, elevated liver enzymes and low platelets
HIV	human immunodeficiency virus
HPV	human papillomavirus
HRT	hormone replacement therapy
HVS	high vaginal swab
IUCD	intrauterine contraceptive device
IUGR	intrauterine growth restriction
IUS	intrauterine system
IV	intravenous
IVF	*in-vitro* fertilization
IVP	intravenous pyelogram
LDL	low-density lipoprotein
LFT	liver function test
LH	luteinizing hormone
LLETZ	large loop excision of the transformation zone
LMP	last menstrual period
LNG-IUS	levonorgestrel intrauterine system
MCV	mean corpuscular volume
MSU	mid-stream specimen of urine
NHS	National Health Service
NICE	National Institute for Health and Clinical Excellence
NIDDM	non-insulin dependent diabetes mellitus
NSAID	non-steroidal anti-inflammatory drug
NTD	neural tube defect
OAB	over active bladder
PCOS	polycystic ovarian syndrome
PE	pulmonary embolism
PID	pelvic inflammatory disease
PR	per rectum
PROM	preterm rupture of the membranes
REM	rapid eye movement
RMI	relative malignancy index
RCOG	Royal College of Obstetricians and Gynaecologists
sb-hCG	serum beta-human chorionic gonadotrophin
SSRIs	selective serotonin reuptake inhibitors
TAH	total abdominal hysterectomy
TCRE	transcervical resection of the endometrium
TDF	testicular development factor
TFT	thyroid function test
TPHA	*Treponema pallidum* haemagglutination assay
TPPA	*Treponema pallidum* particle agglutination
TSH	thyroid-stimulating hormone
TTTS	twin-to-twin transfusion syndrome
TVT	tension-free vaginal tape
U&Es	urea and electrolytes
USI	urodynamic-proven stress incontinence
USS	ultrasound scan
UTI	urinary tract infection
VDRL	Venereal Disease Research Laboratory
VKDB	vitamin K deficiency bleeding
VMA	vanillylmandelic acid
V/Q	ventilation/perfusion
VTE	venous thromboembolism

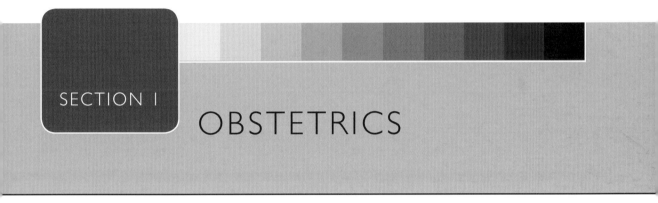

SECTION 1

OBSTETRICS

EXTENDED MATCHING QUESTIONS

QUESTIONS

1 Pre-existing maternal conditions

A Diabetes	E Factor V Leiden deficiency	I Crohn's disease
B Hypertension	F HIV	J Mitral valve stenosis
C Epilepsy	G Asthma	K Myasthenia gravis
D Vitiligo	H Smoking	L Glomerulonephritis

For each description below, choose the SINGLE most appropriate answer from the above list of options. Each option may be used once, more than once, or not at all.

1 Reduces intrauterine growth in a dose-dependent manner.
2 Increases risk of venous thromboembolism (VTE) in the puerperium.
3 Increased frequency of episodes during pregnancy.
4 Risk of fetal macrosomia if condition not well controlled.
5 Maternal muscle fatigue in labour.
6 Requires prophylactic antibiotics for instrumental delivery.

2 Gravidity/parity

A GI P0	**E** G2 PI	**I** GI PI
B G4 P2	**F** GI P2	**J** G3 PI
C G0 P0	**G** G6 P0	**K** G4 P3
D G3 P3	**H** G5 P2	**L** G2 P0

For each description below, choose the SINGLE most appropriate answer from the above list of options. Each option may be used once, more than once, or not at all.

1 A woman currently pregnant who has had a previous term delivery.
2 A woman not currently pregnant who has had one previous termination, one early miscarriage and one still-birth at 36/40.
3 A woman who attends for pre-conception counselling, never having been pregnant.
4 A woman currently pregnant with twins who has had one previous early miscarriage.
5 A woman not currently pregnant who previously had a twin delivery at 28/40.

3 Maternal and perinatal mortality: the confidential enquiry

A Maternal death	**D** Maternal mortality rate	**G** Stillbirth
B Direct maternal death	**E** Perinatal death	**H** None of the above
C Indirect maternal death	**F** Perinatal mortality rate	

For each description below, choose the SINGLE most appropriate answer from the above list of options. Each option may be used once, more than once, or not at all.

1 Death of a woman while pregnant, or within 42 days of termination of pregnancy, from any cause related to, or aggravated by, the pregnancy or its management, but not from accidental or incidental death.
2 The number of stillbirths and early neonatal deaths per 1000 live births and stillbirths.
3 Fetal death occurring between 20 + 0 weeks and 23 + 6 weeks. If the gestation is not certain all births of at least 300 g are reported.
4 Death resulting from previous existing disease, or disease that developed during pregnancy and which was not due to direct obstetric cause, but which was aggravated by the effects of pregnancy that are due to direct or indirect maternal causes.

4 Standards in maternity care

A Royal College of Obstetricians and Gynaecologists	**E** National Childbirth Trust	**I** Maternity Services Liaison Committee
B Clinical Negligence Scheme for Trusts	**F** National Institute for Health and Clinical Excellence	**J** Confidential Enquiry into Maternal and Child Health
C The Cochrane Library	**G** World Health Organization	**K** National Screening Committee
D Maternity Matters	**H** National Library for Health	**L** National Health Service

For each description below, choose the SINGLE most appropriate answer from the above list of options. Each option may be used once, more than once, or not at all.

1 Publishes national guidelines on all aspects of clinical care, including obstetric practice.
2 National consumer group representing the views of women on maternity care.
3 Sets standards for provision of care, training and revalidation of obstetric doctors in the UK.
4 An insurance scheme to help hospital Trusts fund ligation claims and manage risk.
5 Unifies and progresses standards for screening across the UK.

5 Physiological changes in pregnancy: uterus and cervix

A Oestradiol
B Prostaglandins
C Progesterone
D Cortisol

E Collagenase
F Prolactin
G Human chorionic
   gonadotrophin (HCG)

H Adrenocorticotrophic hormone
   (ACTH)
I Oxytocin

For each description below, choose the SINGLE most appropriate answer from the above list of options. Each option may be used once, more than once, or not at all.

1 Levels approximately x15 higher in third trimester than in non-pregnant state.
2 Induces the process of cervical remodelling.
3 Regulates local uterine blood flow through endothelial effects.
4 Utilized in triple test.
5 Released from posterior pituitary gland.

6 Haematological changes in pregnancy

A Haematocrit
B Bilirubin
C Triglycerides

D Plasma folate concentration
E White blood cells
F Tissue plasminogen activator

G Fibrinogen
H Alkaline phosphatase
I Lactate dehydrogenase

For each description below, choose the SINGLE most appropriate answer from the above list of options. Each option may be used once, more than once, or not at all.

1 Levels rise through pregnancy due to increased production of placental isoform.
2 Falls in pregnancy due to dilutional effect.
3 Increased by 50 per cent in pregnancy, contributing to hypercoagulable state.
4 Routine supplementation advised during pregnancy due to fall in level.

7 Normal fetal development: the fetal heart

A The ductus venosus
B The ductus arteriosus
C Foramen ovale
D Left atrium

E Right atrium
F Mitral valve
G Tricuspid valve
H Umbilical vein

I Umbilical artery
J Atrial septum
K Intraventricular septum
L None of the above

For each description below, choose the SINGLE most appropriate answer from the above list of options. Each option may be used once, more than once, or not at all.

1 Location of the patent foramen ovale.
2 Vessel that carries oxygenated blood from the placenta and, in adult life, forms part of the falciform ligament.
3 Connects the pulmonary artery to the descending aorta.
4 Vessel that shunts blood away from the liver.

8 Normal fetal development: the urinary tract

A Mesonephric duct
B Glomeruli
C Ureteric bud

D Collecting duct system
E Ectoderm
F Mesoderm

G Nephronic units
H Renal agenesis
I Pronephros

For each description below, choose the SINGLE most appropriate answer from the above list of options. Each option may be used once, more than once, or not at all.

1 Originates on either side of the embryonic midline on the nephrogenic ridge.
2 Branches to form the collecting duct system.
3 Associated with anhydramnios and neonatal death.
4 Embryonic layer from which the renal parenchyma is derived.

9 Antenatal care

A Triple test	**E** Dating scan	**I** Biophysical profile
B Ferritin	**F** Syphilis	**J** Anatomy scan
C Mid-stream urine specimen	**G** Protein dip stick	**K** Nuchal translucency
D Full blood count (FBC)	**H** Serum urate	

For each description below, choose the SINGLE most appropriate answer from the above list of options. Each option may be used once, more than once, or not at all.

1 Second trimester screening for Down's syndrome.
2 A fetal viability test.
3 A screening test for pre-eclampsia.
4 Should routinely be performed at booking and repeated at 28/40.

10 NICE guidelines on routine antenatal care

A Booking visit	**E** 25/40	**I** 36/40
B 10–14/40	**F** 28/40	**J** 38/40
C 16/40	**G** 31/40	**K** 40/40
D 18–20/40	**H** 34/40	**L** 41/40

For each description below, choose the SINGLE most appropriate answer from the above list of options. Each option may be used once, more than once, or not at all.

1 Attend for ultrasound to detect structural abnormalities.
2 Folic acid and lifestyle issues discussed.
3 Offer membrane sweep.
4 First dose of anti-D prophylaxis for Rhesus –ve women.

11 Antenatal imaging and assessment of fetal well-being

A Variable decelerations	**E** Fetal heart rate accelerations	**I** Biophysical profile
B Late decelerations	**F** Antenatal Doppler	**J** None of the above
C Early decelerations	**G** Doppler in labour	
D Baseline variability	**H** Diagnostic ultrasound	

For each description below, choose the SINGLE most appropriate answer from the above list of options. Each option may be used once, more than once, or not at all.

1 Reflection of the normal fetal autonomic nervous system.
2 Assessment of fetal breathing, gross body movements, fetal tone, reactive fetal heart rate and amniotic fluid.
3 Transient reduction in the fetal heart rate of 15 beats per minute or more, lasting for more than 15 seconds.
4 Transient increase in the fetal heart rate of 15 beats per minute or more, lasting for more than 15 seconds.

12 Ultrasound measurements

A Crown–rump length
B Biparietal diameter (BPD)
C Estimated fetal weight
D Head circumference (HC)
E Femur length (FL)
F HC/AC ratio
G Abdominal circumference (AC)
H Placental site
I Nuchal translucency

For each description below, choose the SINGLE most appropriate answer from the above list of options. Each option may be used once, more than once, or not at all.

1 Used to date pregnancies when booked between 14 and 20/40.
2 Marker of asymmetrical intrauterine growth restriction (IUGR).
3 Increased in infants of poorly controlled diabetic mothers.
4 Can be calculated by combining HC/AC/FL(femur length)/BPD measurements.

13 Prenatal diagnosis

A Spina bifida
B Down's syndrome
C Duchenne muscular dystrophy
D Thalassaemia
E Cerebral palsy
F Klinefelter's syndrome
G Turner's syndrome
H Fragile X
I None of the above

For each description below, choose the SINGLE most appropriate answer from the above list of options. Each option may be used once, more than once, or not at all.

1 The diagnosis may be suspected on ultrasound where enlargement of the ventricles is observed.
2 Ultrasound between 11 and 14 weeks in combination with blood tests is a reliable method of screening.
3 Prenatal diagnosis is available by the demonstration of multiple repeats (>200) in a male fetus.
4 Affected individuals are infertile males, some of whom have reduced intelligence, testicular dysgenesis and tall stature.

14 Modes of prenatal testing

A Amniocentesis
B Viral serology
C Nuchal translucency
D Ultrasound scan
E Cordocentesis
F Fetal RNA profile
G Chorionic villus sampling (CVS)
H Free fetal DNA
I None of the above

For each description below, choose the SINGLE most appropriate answer from the above list of options. Each option may be used once, more than once, or not at all.

1 Most suitable diagnostic test where a woman wishes to know fetal karyotype as early in the pregnancy as possible.
2 Most suitable diagnostic test where fetal alloimmune thrombocytopaenia is suspected.
3 Most suitable non-invasive test when an X-linked disorder is suspected.
4 Non-invasive test which will give a reliable diagnosis of a fetal single gene defect.

15 Antepartum haemorrhage

A Placenta praevia
B Placental abruption
C Rectal bleeding
D Threatened preterm labour
E Vasa praevia
F Cancer of the cervix
G Vaginal infection
H Cervical trauma
I None of the above

For each description below, choose the SINGLE most appropriate answer from the above list of options. Each option may be used once, more than once, or not at all.

1   A 32-year-old woman presented to the delivery suite. She was 28 weeks pregnant in her second pregnancy. An ultrasound scan at 12 weeks had confirmed a twin pregnancy. She was admitted complaining of bleeding per vaginum; this was bright red in nature and painless.

2   A 36-year-old woman presented to the delivery with a small amount of fresh red vaginal bleeding. She was 36 weeks pregnant with her third child. She was in no pain and speculum examination revealed a trace of bright red blood in the vagina. She had a history of sexual intercourse 4 hours earlier.

3   A 19-year-old woman presented to the emergency department with a small amount of blood-stained discharge. She was 30 weeks into her first pregnancy. Speculum examination revealed thick off-white discharge mixed with a little brownish blood in the vagina.

4   A 32-year-old woman presented to the delivery suite. She was 34 weeks pregnant in her first pregnancy. She was admitted complaining of severe abdominal pain, and bright red bleeding and clots per vaginum. On examination, the uterus was painful and there were palpable contractions.

16 Fetal malpresentations

A   Transverse
B   Frank breech
C   Extended breech
D   Footling breech
E   Cephalic
F   Oblique
G   Unstable lie
H   Complete breech
I   None of the above

For each description below, choose the SINGLE most appropriate answer from the above list of options. Each option may be used once, more than once, or not at all.

1   Longitudinal lie where the presenting part is a foot.
2   The fetal long axis runs perpendicular to the maternal long axis.
3   Women should routinely be admitted to the antenatal ward at term.
4   The position intended to be achieved by external cephalic version.

17 Thromboprophylaxis

A   No intervention required
B   Lifelong anticoagulation
C   Intravenous (IV) unfractionated heparin for 24 hours
D   6 weeks post-natal low molecular weight heparin
E   Discussion with haematologist for expert advice
F   1 week post-natal low molecular weight heparin
G   Early mobilization and hydration
H   Antenatal prophylaxis with low molecular weight heparin
I   None of the above

For each description below, choose the SINGLE most appropriate answer from the above list of options. Each option may be used once, more than once, or not at all.

1   A woman attends for booking at 6 weeks of pregnancy. She has had a previous metallic mitral valve replacement.
2   A 28-year-old woman who has had an emergency Caesarean section in labour for fetal distress. She had a DVT in a previous pregnancy.
3   A healthy 30-year-old woman had a normal vaginal delivery of her fourth child 4 hours ago.
4   A healthy 36-year-old woman had a normal vaginal delivery of her fourth child 4 hours ago.

18 Common problems of pregnancy

A Constipation
B Oedema
C Leg cramps
D Fainting

E Leg cramps
F Hyperemesis gravidarum
G Breast soreness
H Symphysis pubis dysfunction

I Striae gravidarum
J Carpal tunnel syndrome
K Tiredness
L Gastro-oesophageal reflux

For each description below, choose the SINGLE most appropriate answer from the above list of options. Each option may be used once, more than once, or not at all.

1 Best treated with simple analgesia and low stability belt.
2 Due to hormonal effects in relaxing the lower oesophageal sphincter.
3 Hydration and use of compression stockings may help to prevent.
4 May be exacerbated by administration of iron tablets.

19 Twins and higher order multiple gestations

A Miscarriage
B Dichorionic diamniotic twins
C Monochorionic monoamniotic twins
D Twin–twin transfusion syndrome

E Preterm labour
F Nuchal translucency
G Triple test
H Monochorionic diamniotic twins
I Pre-eclampsia

J Monozygotic twins
K None of the above

For each description below, choose the SINGLE most appropriate answer from the above list of options. Each option may be used once, more than once, or not at all.

1 The observation of the lambda sign on early ultrasound confirms the diagnosis.
2 Death or handicap of the co-twin occurs in 25 per cent of cases.
3 Result of single embryo splitting between 4 and 8 days post-fertilization.
4 Imbalance in blood flow across placental vascular anastomoses.

20 Management of multiple pregnancy

A Fortnightly ultrasound scans
B Ultrasound measurement of cervical length
C Internal podalic version

D Lambda sign
E Elective Caesarean section at 36–37 weeks
F Multi-fetal reduction

G Maternal steroid therapy
H 4–6-weekly ultrasound scans
I Elective Caesarean section at 32–34 weeks

For each description below, choose the SINGLE most appropriate answer from the above list of options. Each option may be used once, more than once, or not at all.

1 Recommended surveillance for monozygotic twins in the third trimester.
2 May be considered in higher order multiple pregnancies to reduce the possibility of preterm birth.
3 Helpful in predicting preterm labour in multiple pregnancies.
4 Most common delivery strategy for monozygotic monoamniotic twins.

21 The clinical management of hypertension in pregnancy

A   Magnesium hydroxide
B   Oral antihypertensive
C   Oral diuretic
D   Outpatient monitoring of blood pressure

E   Renal function tests
F   24-hour urine protein collection
G   Admission for observation and investigation
H   Fetal ultrasound

I   Immediate Caesarean section
J   Induction of labour
K   Intravenous antihypertensives
L   None of the above

For each description below, choose the SINGLE most appropriate answer from the above list of options. Each option may be used once, more than once, or not at all.

1   At 34 weeks, an 80 kg woman complains of persistent headaches and 'flashing lights'. There is no hyper-reflexia and her blood pressure (BP) is 155/90 mmHg.

2   At 33 weeks, a 31-year-old primigravida is found to have BP of 145/95 mmHg. At her first visit at 12 weeks, the BP was 145/85 mmHg. She has no proteinuria but she is found to have oedema to her knees. Her renal function tests are normal.

3   A 29-year-old woman has an uneventful first pregnancy to 31 weeks. She is then admitted as an emergency with epigastric pain. During the first 3 hours, her BP rises from 150/100 to 170/119 mmHg. A dipstick test reveals she has 3+ proteinuria. The fetal cardiotocogram is normal.

4   A 32-year-old woman in her second pregnancy presents to her general practitioner (GP) at 12 weeks' gestation. She was mildly hypertensive in her previous pregnancy. Her BP is 150/100 mmHg; 2 weeks later, at the hospital antenatal clinic, her BP is 155/100 mmHg.

22 Features of abnormal placentation

A   HELLP syndrome
B   Pre-eclampsia
C   Eclampsia

D   Disseminated intravascular coagulation
E   Glomeruloendotheliosis
F   Gestational hypertension

G   Chronic hypertension
H   Placental abruption
I   None of the above

For each description below, choose the SINGLE most appropriate answer from the above list of options. Each option may be used once, more than once, or not at all.

1   A 40-year-old woman in her first pregnancy presents in labour. Her blood pressure is 145/90. Shortly after beginning regular contractions she has a tonic-clonic seizure.

2   A 32-year-old woman presents at 38/40 in her second pregnancy, her first having been complicated by pre-eclampsia. Her blood pressure is 130/85 and her alanine amino transferase (ALT) is 70.

3   A 24-year-old woman in her first pregnancy presents at 32/40 with sudden onset severe abdominal pain and vaginal bleeding. Her blood pressure is 160/95.

4   A 36-year-old woman in her first pregnancy is noted to have a blood pressure of 140/85 at 32/40. There is no protein in her urine and she is asymptomatic.

23 Late miscarriage

A   Threatened miscarriage
B   Inevitable miscarriage
C   Missed miscarriage

D   Stillbirth
E   Complete miscarriage
F   Chorioamnionitis

G   Urinary tract infection
H   None of the above

For each description below, choose the SINGLE most appropriate answer from the above list of options. Each option may be used once, more than once, or not at all.

1 A 23-year-old woman presents at 21/40. She is complaining of low backache and suprapubic discomfort. Routine examination of the patient's abdomen reveals that there is suprapubic tenderness. Examination of her vital signs reveals pyrexia of 37.7°C and a tachycardia of 90 beats per minute. Internal examination reveals that the cervix is closed. Urine dipstick demonstrates leukocytes and nitrites.

2 A 23-year-old woman presents at 23/40 in her second pregnancy. The first pregnancy had unfortunately ended at 19 weeks with a miscarriage after premature rupture of the fetal membranes. She is complaining of low backache, feeling hot and a slight vaginal loss. She has pyrexia of 38°C and a pulse of 98 beats per minute. Routine examination of the patient's abdomen reveals that there is tenderness suprapubically. Speculum examination reveals a slightly open cervix and fluid draining.

3 A 23-year-old woman presents at 21/40. She is complaining of vaginal bleeding, low backache and suprapubic discomfort. Routine examination of the patient's abdomen reveals that there is suprapubic tenderness. Examination of her vital signs demonstrates that she is apyrexial. Internal examination reveals that the cervix is closed. Urine dipstick is unremarkable.

4 A 32-year-old woman presents in her first pregnancy at 20 weeks of amenorrhoea. She is complaining of minor discomfort in the lower abdomen. Her pulse and blood pressure are within the normal range and she is apyrexial. Abdominal examination is unremarkable. However, speculum examination reveals a slightly open cervix. A transvaginal ultrasound scan demonstrates the cervical canal to be 2 cm long and funnelling of the membranes is present.

24 Risk factors for preterm labour

A Smoking
B Uterine abnormality
C Appendicitis
D Parity >5
E Previous preterm delivery
F Intrauterine bleeding
G Cervical fibroids
H Poor socioeconomic background
I Interpregnancy interval <one year
J Afro-Caribbean origin
K Multiple pregnancy
L Previous cervical cone biopsy

For each description below, choose the SINGLE most appropriate answer from the above list of options. Each option may be used once, more than once, or not at all.

1 Risk of preterm labour is primarily due to uterine over-distension.
2 Linked to recurrent episodes of threatened miscarriage early in pregnancy.
3 May require surgery during pregnancy with associated risk of preterm labour.
4 Modifiable risk factor for which help and advice can be given in antenatal clinic.

25 Diagnosis and management of preterm delivery

A Fetal fibronectin testing
B Maternal steroids
C Cardiotocography (CTG) monitoring
D Cervical length measurement
E Nitrazine test
F Cervical cerclage
G Amniocentesis
H Tocolysis
I High vaginal swabs

For each description below, choose the SINGLE most appropriate answer from the above list of options. Each option may be used once, more than once, or not at all.

1 High negative predictive value for detecting preterm pre-labour rupture of the membranes.
2 May allow a window of opportunity for antenatal steroid administration or intrauterine transfer.
3 Contraindicated in the presence of vaginal bleeding, contractions or infection.
4 Invasive test for chorioamnionitis.

26 Drugs used in pregnancy

A Calcium supplements	**D** Ritodrine	**G** Oral labetolol
B Erythromycin	**E** Ursodeoxycholic acid	**H** Ferrous sulphate
C Nifedipine	**F** Magnesium sulphate	**I** None of the above

For each description below, choose the SINGLE most appropriate drug treatment from the above list of options. Each option may be used once, more than once, or not at all.

1 A 27-year-old woman presents at 33 weeks in her first pregnancy. She is complaining of generalized itching, worse on the palms of her hands and soles of her feet. Abdominal examination is unremarkable. Blood investigations reveal that she has increased bile acids.

2 A 23-year-old primigravid woman presents at 31 weeks. At her 12-weeks booking visit she was normotensive and had no history of epilepsy. She is admitted as an emergency having had a seizure. On admission, her blood pressure is 150/110 mmHg and dipstick urine analysis reveals 3+ proteinuria.

3 A 32-year-old woman presents in her second pregnancy at 29 weeks. Her first pregnancy had been uncomplicated; however, she had delivered at 36 weeks' gestation. She is admitted with a history of sudden gush of fluid per vaginum. On examination her abdomen is consistent with a 29-week pregnancy. Speculum examination reveals copious amounts of clear fluid. Temperature and pulse are normal.

4 A 25-year-old Asian woman in her third pregnancy presents to clinic at 24 weeks of her pregnancy. She is complaining of tiredness and lethargy. Abdominal examination is unremarkable. Dipstick urine analysis demonstrates 3+ glycosuria. A full blood count reveals haemoglobin of 11 g/dL. An oral glucose tolerance test shows a fasting blood glucose of 8.1 mmol/L.

27 Shortness of breath in pregnancy

A Pneumonia	**D** Cystic fibrosis	**G** Mitral stenosis
B Ischaemic heart disease	**E** Pulmonary embolism	**H** Pulmonary hypertension
C Asthma	**F** Ventricular septal defect	**I** None of the above

For each description below, choose the SINGLE most appropriate answer from the above list of options. Each option may be used once, more than once, or not at all.

1 At least 30 per cent of women show an improvement in the condition during pregnancy and there is no increased risk of exacerbation postpartum.

2 Requires close attention to nutritional status, physiotherapy and treatment of infections in pregnancy.

3 Patients should be strongly advised against pregnancy, due to high risk of maternal mortality.

4 40 per cent experience worsening symptoms in pregnancy, with a risk of pulmonary oedema in the third trimester.

28 Perinatal infection (1)

A Toxoplasmosis	**E** *Listeria monocytogenes*	**I** *Neisseria gonorrhoeae*
B Cytomegalovirus	**F** Parvovirus	**J** Trichomoniasis
C *Varicella zoster*	**G** *Chlamydia trachomatis*	**K** *Yersinia pestis*
D Cocksackie B virus	**H** Group B streptococcus	**L** None of the above

For each description below, choose the SINGLE most appropriate answer from the above list of options. Each option may be used once, more than once, or not at all.

1 A bacterium that is found in sewage, but can grow in refrigerated food, including meat, eggs and dairy products.
2 A protozoan parasite that may be acquired from exposure to cat faeces or from eating uncooked meats.
3 In children it causes a viral exanthema known as 'fifth disease'.
4 Primary infection usually presents within 7 days of exposure and may be accompanied by wide lesions around the vulva, vagina and cervix.

29 Perinatal infection (2)

A HIV
B Hepatitis C
C Plasmodium falciparum
D Varicella zoster
E Treponema pallidum
F Recurrent genital herpes infection
G Rubella
H Hepatitis B
I None of the above

For each description below, choose the SINGLE most appropriate answer from the above list of options. Each option may be used once, more than once, or not at all.

1 Delivery by elective Caesarean section may decrease transmission rate.
2 Immunity is 90 per cent in the UK adult population.
3 Treatment may provoke a Jarisch–Herxheimer reaction.
4 Vaccination during pregnancy is contraindicated, but should be given after pregnancy if non-immune.

30 Mechanism of labour

A Descent
B Extension
C Engagement
D Flexion
E External rotation
F Restitution
G Internal rotation
H None of the above

For each description below, choose the SINGLE most appropriate answer from the above list of options. Each option may be used once, more than once, or not at all.

1 After the head delivers through the vulva, it immediately aligns with the fetal shoulders.
2 The occiput escapes from underneath the symphysis pubis, which acts as a fulcrum.
3 The anterior shoulder lies inferior to the symphysis pubis and delivers first, and the posterior shoulder delivers subsequently.
4 When the widest part of the presenting part has passed successfully through the pelvic inlet.

31 Stages of labour

A Latent phase
B Third stage
C Transition
D Passive descent
E First stage
F Braxton-Hicks contractions
G Effacement
H Active second stage
I None of the above

For each description below, choose the SINGLE most appropriate answer from the above list of options. Each option may be used once, more than once, or not at all.

1 Should be considered abnormal if lasting more than 30 minutes.
2 The cervix shortens in length until it becomes included in the lower segment of the uterus.
3 Conventionally should last no longer than 2 hours in a primiparous woman.
4 Time between onset of labour and 3–4 cm cervical dilatation.

32 Interventions in the second stage

A Episiotomy	**D** Syntocinon post-delivery	**G** Kiwi Omnicup
B Metal cup ventouse	**E** Kielland's forceps	**H** Neville Barnes forceps
C Emergency Caesarean	**F** Silicone rubber ventouse cup	**I** None of the above

For each description below, choose the SINGLE most appropriate answer from the above list of options. Each option may be used once, more than once, or not at all.

1 A primigravida in spontaneous labour at 34+3/40 has a pathological trace in the second stage. The fetal head is at +2 station and is occipito-anterior.
2 A multigravida has been induced at 42/40. She has been diagnosed with a brow presentation in the second stage.
3 A primigravida in spontaneous labour at 39+2/40 has been actively pushing for 30 minutes. The fetal head is at 0 station, occipito-transverse.
4 A primigravida in spontaneous labour at 39+2/40 has been actively pushing for 2 hours and is exhausted. The fetal head is at +2 station, occipito-transverse.

33 Complications of Caesarean section

A Pulmonary embolus	**D** Bladder trauma	**G** Bowel injury
B Wound infection	**E** Endometritis	**H** Ileus
C Caesarean hysterectomy	**F** Uterine atony	**I** None of the above

For each description below, choose the SINGLE most appropriate answer from the above list of options. Each option may be used once, more than once, or not at all.

1 A 34-year-old woman who underwent Caesarean section 24 hours ago complains of abdominal pain and distension. Her vital signs are all stable.
2 A 34-year-old woman who underwent Caesarean section 3 days ago complains of severe abdominal pain and distension. She is tachycardic and febrile.
3 A 38-year-old woman who underwent Caesarean section 24 hours ago complains of sharp pain in the shoulder tip and pain on deep inspiration. Her vital signs are stable.
4 A 42-year-old woman who underwent Caesarean section 48 hours ago is diagnosed with the condition that is the leading cause of maternal mortality.

34 Obstetric emergencies (1)

A Simple faint	**D** Pulmonary embolism	**G** Hypoglycaemia
B Epileptic fit	**E** Eclampsia	**H** Ectopic pregnancy
C Subarachnoid haemorrhage	**F** Haemorrhage	**I** None of the above

For each description below, choose the SINGLE most appropriate diagnosis from the above list of options. Each option may be used once, more than once, or not at all.

1 A 37-year-old woman in her second pregnancy has delivered a live male infant. She has no medical history of note. 10 minutes after delivery, she complains of a sudden onset severe occipital headache that is associated with vomiting. Shortly after this, she loses consciousness and is unresponsive to any stimuli.
2 A 23-year-old woman who is 32 weeks pregnant presents to delivery suite. She complains of feeling generally unwell. Clinical examination reveals a 28-week size fetus. Her blood pressure was noted to be 120/90 mmHg and on urine analysis 2+ protein was present. During the clinical examination, she has a seizure.

3 A 32-year-old woman who has had an emergency Caesarean section is on the post-natal ward. She suddenly becomes breathless and complains of central chest pain. She subsequently loses consciousness.

35 Obstetric emergencies (2)

A Cord prolapse
B Amniotic fluid embolus
C HELLP syndrome
D Uterine atony
E Pulmonary embolus
F Uterine inversion
G Uterine rupture
H Eclamptic seizure
I Shoulder dystocia

For each description below, choose the SINGLE most appropriate diagnosis from the above list of options. Each option may be used once, more than once, or not at all.

1 A 38-year-old gestational diabetic with a BMI of 35 is induced at 42/40. After a long labour, the obstetric registrar plans to deliver with forceps.
2 A 27-year-old woman is admitted with spontaneous rupture of the membranes and mild contractions at 30/40. An ultrasound examination reveals the fetus to be in a footling breech position.
3 A 34-year-old woman is fully dilated and pushing during her second labour. Her contractions have been augmented with syntocinon. Her first child was born by emergency Caesarean.
4 After delivery, a 36-year-old woman has failed to complete the third stage. The obstetrician is anxious to avoid taking her to theatre.

36 Postpartum pyrexia

A Pyelonephritis
B Mastitis
C Pneumonia
D Deep vein thrombosis
E Meningitis
F Endometritis
G Wound infection
H Retained products of conception
I Breast abscess
J Chest infection
K None of the above

For each description below, choose the SINGLE most appropriate answer from the above list of options. Each option may be used once, more than once, or not at all.

1 A 30-year-old woman is admitted from home. She had an uncomplicated pregnancy and a normal vaginal delivery 4 days previously. She presented with feeling generally unwell associated with heavy, fresh vaginal bleeding and clots. On examination, she has a temperature of 38.3°C. Abdominal examination reveals mild suprapubic tenderness. Vaginal examination reveals blood clots and the cervix admits a finger and is enlarged and bulky.
2 A 26-year-old woman is admitted 7 days after having a Caesarean section, which was performed for failure to progress after augmentation for prolonged rupture of the fetal membranes. She is generally unwell and complains of a foul-smelling vaginal discharge. On examination, she has a temperature of 39.0°C. Abdominal examination reveals suprapubic tenderness. Vaginal examination confirms the offensive discharge and uterine tenderness.
3 A 32-year-old woman is seen 3 days after having a Caesarean section. The Caesarean section was performed as an emergency for placental abruption and was carried out under general anaesthesia. She is complaining that she is generally unwell and has been coughing up green sputum. On examination, she has a temperature of 38.0°C and a pulse of 90 beats per minute. The respiratory rate is 30 inspirations per minute and she is using her accessory respiratory muscles. Abdominal and pelvic examinations are unremarkable. Chest examination reveals purulent sputum and coarse crackles of auscultation.

37 Postpartum contraception

A   Oral contraceptive pill
B   Postpartum amenorrhoea and
    full breastfeeding
C   Progesterone-only pill

D   Depo-provera
E   Sterilization at Caesarean
    section
F   Condoms

G   Laparoscopic clip sterilization
H   Intrauterine contraceptive
    device
I   None of the above

For each description below, choose the SINGLE most appropriate diagnosis from the above list of options. Each option may be used once, more than once, or not at all.

1   4–8 weeks for uterine involution before utilizing.
2   Gives less than 2 per cent chance of conceiving in first six months.
3   Lowest failure rate in ensuring no further pregnancies are possible.
4   Increases risk of thromboembolism in the puerperium.

38 Psychiatric disorders in pregnancy and the puerperium

A   Baby blues
B   Post-natal depression
C   Panic disorders

D   Schizophrenia
E   Puerperal psychosis
F   Bipolar affective disorder

G   Depression
H   Post-natal 'pinks'
I   None of the above

For each description below, choose the SINGLE most appropriate answer from the above list of options. Each option may be used once, more than once, or not at all.

1   A 40-year-old woman presents on the fifth day after a normal delivery. Her husband has brought her into accident and emergency after he noticed an abrupt change in her behaviour. He describes her as confused, restless and expressing thoughts of self-harm.
2   A 23-year-old woman, who had a normal delivery 24 hours earlier, is noted by the ward staff to be having difficulties sleeping and expresses feelings of excitement.
3   A 23-year-old woman presents at a booking clinic. She is 7 weeks pregnant in her first pregnancy and has been referred by the community midwife for consultant care. She is taking lithium and carbamazepine.
4   A 32-year-old woman who had an emergency Caesarean section 2 days earlier is noted by the midwives on the ward to be having sleeping difficulties and is tearful and short-tempered.

39 Neonatology

A   Erythema toxicum
B   Erb's palsy
C   Klumpke's palsy
D   Necrotizing enterocolitis
E   Subgaleal haemorrhage

F   Transient tachypnoea of the
    newborn
G   Respiratory distress syndrome
H   Cerebral palsy
I   Milia

J   Port wine stain
K   None of the above

For each description below, choose the SINGLE most appropriate answer from the above list of options. Each option may be used once, more than once, or not at all.

1   A newborn baby of 36 weeks' gestation presents with cyanosis, tachypnoea, grunting and recession.
2   In a newborn post-natal check of a term baby delivered by vaginal breech, the attending senior house officer (SHO) notices that there is a claw hand with inability to extend the fingers.
3   The senior house officer is asked to review a 3-day-old baby. The baby has an oval erythematous rash with white pinpoint heads.

40 Neonatal care

A Special care
B Paediatrician at delivery
C High-dependency care
D Care on post-natal ward
E Maximal intensive care
F Full septic screen
G Suitable for early discharge
H Phototherapy
I None of the above

For each description below, choose the SINGLE most appropriate answer from the above list of options. Each option may be used once, more than once, or not at all.

1 A male infant was delivered 24 hours ago at 28+3/40 in the breech position. His mother had a history of preterm delivery.
2 A female infant was delivered 16 hours ago at 37/40, weighing 4.1 kg. Her mother had poorly controlled gestational diabetes.
3 A 35-year-old primigravida is in spontaneous labour at 37+1/40 with dichorionic diamniotic twins.
4 A male infant was delivered 3 days ago at 34/40. His birthweight was on the 50th centile and septic screen negative, but he continues to have apnoeic attacks.
5 A female infant was delivered 24 hours ago at 39/40 in good condition. Her mother has a long history of psychiatric illness.

41 Neonatal screening

A Neuroblastoma
B Congenital cardiac anomaly
C Phenylketonuria
D Hypoglycaemia
E Hip dysplasia
F Thalassaemia
G Hypothyroidism
H Group B streptococcus
I None of the above

For each description below, choose the SINGLE most appropriate answer from the above list of options. Each option may be used once, more than once, or not at all.

1 All breech babies should undergo screening at 6 weeks old.
2 Overall incidence of 1 in 13 000 babies.
3 Screening test available but trials have shown to be not cost effective for all babies.
4 Developmental delay is significantly reduced if treatment is commenced before 28 days of life.

EMQ ANSWERS

1 Pre-existing maternal conditions

| 1 H | 2 E | 3 C | 4 A | 5 K | 6 J |

Many pre-existing maternal conditions have an impact during pregnancy. Factor V Leiden deficiency increases the risk of venous thromboembolism throughout life and compounds the normal increase in risk in the puerperium. Women with epilepsy often suffer from increased fit frequency during pregnancy. Diabetes can lead to a number of perinatal complications, including fetal macrosomia. Myasthenia gravis can increase the normal maternal muscle fatigue during the course of labour. Women with congenital heart valve problems should have antibiotic prophylaxis for infection-prone procedures such as instrumental delivery.

See Chapter 1, *Obstetrics by Ten Teachers*, 19th edition.

2 Gravidity/Parity

| 1 E | 2 J | 3 C | 4 L | 5 F |

The term 'gravida' describes the total number of pregnancies that a woman has had, regardless of how they ended. The total includes any current pregnancy. The term 'parity' describes the number of live births at any gestation or the number of stillbirths after 24/40. In describing multiple gestations, twins will count as one pregnancy but two live births.

See Chapter 1, *Obstetrics by Ten Teachers*, 19th edition.

3 Maternal and perinatal mortality: the confidential enquiry

| 1 A | 2 F | 3 H | 4 C |

The classification of maternal deaths is a challenge. Data may be collected up to a year after pregnancy for all causes of death, but this is difficult in countries where data collection systems are not well established. ICD 10 (International Classification of Diseases, World Health Organization (WHO)) defines maternal death by the definition given in part 1. Numbers expressed as events per 1000 of the relevant population are rates. The definition given in part 3 relates to late fetal loss and hence does not fit with any of the answers given.

See Chapter 2, *Obstetrics by Ten Teachers*, 19th edition.

4 Standards in maternity care

| 1 F | 2 E | 3 A | 4 B | 5 K |

The National Institute for Health and Clinical Excellence publishes UK guidelines in all clinical specialties. The National Childbirth Trust is an influential consumer group in the UK, represented on many panels and committees. The Royal College of Obstetricians and Gynaecologists (RCOG) defines standards for training obstetricians and gynaecologists among many other roles. The Clinical Negligence Scheme for Trusts provides a means for trusts to cope with potentially extremely high obstetric litigation bills, and incentivizes good clinical care.

See Chapter 2, *Obstetrics by Ten Teachers*, 19th edition.

5 Physiological changes in pregnancy: uterus and cervix

1 F   2 B   3 D   4 G   5 I

Prolactin is produced by the anterior pituitary gland and is essential for the stimulation of milk secretion. The levels of prolactin are increased 15-fold during late pregnancy. Cervical remodelling is induced by prostaglandins (used clinically for this indication). Local collagenase release also aids in cervical softening. Maternal cortisol regulates uterine blood flow through effects on vascular endothelium and smooth muscle. Beta human chorionic gonadotrophin is one of the components of the triple test, with alpha-fetoprotein and oestriol. Oxytocin and antidiuretic hormone (ADH) are the clinically significant hormones released from the posterior pituitary.

See Chapter 3, *Obstetrics by Ten Teachers*, 19th edition.

6 Haematological changes in pregnancy

1 H   2 A   3 G   4 D

Alkaline phosphatase has isoforms from a number of organs, including liver and bone. The placental isoform accounts for the dramatic rise in late pregnancy. Although the erythrocyte mass increases in pregnancy, haematocrit falls due to the proportionally larger increase in plasma volume. The majority of procoagulant factors, including fibrinogen, are increased during pregnancy. This accounts in part for the 5-fold increase in incidence of venous thromboembolism in pregnancy, but also helps to prevent major haemorrhage at placental separation. Folate supplementation is currently advised for all pregnant women in an attempt to reduce the incidence of neural tube defects (NTDs).

See Chapter 3, *Obstetrics by Ten Teachers*, 19th edition.

7 Normal fetal development: the fetal heart

1 J   2 H   3 B   4 A

The adaptations of the cardiovascular system at birth comprise the loss of the low-resistance placental shunt and the addition of the pulmonary circulation in parallel to the systemic. This requires closure of the foramen ovale, located in the atrial septum. Oxygenated blood travels from the placenta towards the fetal heart in the umbilical vein. The ductus arteriosus connects the pulmonary artery to the descending aorta *in utero* forming the ligamentum arteriosum at birth. Blood is shunted from the umbilical vein to the vena cava, bypassing the liver by the ductus venosus.

See Chapter 4, *Obstetrics by Ten Teachers*, 19th edition.

8 Normal fetal development: the urinary tract

1 I   2 C   3 H   4 F

The fetal urinary tract has one of the more complicated embryological origins. It is preceded by two primitive forms, the pronephros and the mesonephros. The pronephros originates at about 3 weeks as the nephrogenic ridge either side of the midline. The ureteric bud is the origin of the collecting duct system. The renal parenchyma derives from the mesonephric tubules, which are composed from mesoderm tissue. After 16 weeks the fetal kidneys are responsible for amniotic fluid production and hence renal agenesis will result in anhydramnios.

See Chapter 4, *Obstetrics by Ten Teachers*, 19th edition.

9 Antenatal care

1 A   2 E   3 G   4 D

The triple test consists of beta human chorionic gonadotrophin, alpha-fetoprotein and oestriol. In many areas it has been superseded by nuchal translucency in combination with biochemical tests. The dating scan has several specific aims, which include fetal viability, dating, diagnosis and chorionicity of twins. Assessment of proteinuria with blood pressure measurement is the main screening test for pre-eclampsia. It is usual to take a full blood count at booking and at 28 weeks.

See Chapter 5, *Obstetrics by Ten Teachers*, 19th edition.

10 NICE guidelines on routine antenatal care

1 D   2 A   3 L   4 F

The fetal anomaly scan is usually scheduled between 18 and 22 weeks. This timing allows for early pregnancy loss and gives sufficient time for morphogenesis, while allowing information on abnormalities to be available to patients as early as possible. Folic acid and lifestyle issues should be discussed as early in pregnancy as possible, usually at the booking visit. A membrane sweep is offered in normal pregnancy at 41 weeks in an attempt to avoid induction for post-date pregnancy. Anti-D prophylaxis is usually given routinely at 28/40 and 34/40.

See Chapter 5, *Obstetrics by Ten Teachers*, 19th edition.

11 Antenatal imaging and assessment of fetal well-being

1 D   2 I   3 J   4 E

The cardiotocograph (CTG) comprises a continuous tracing of the fetal heart. Specific features of this tracing are sought to help clinicians assess potential concern regarding fetal well-being in utero. Baseline variability is affected by physiological conditions and reflects the fetal autonomic system. It may therefore be altered by conditions including fetal sleep cycles and maternal drug administration. A deceleration on a CTG is defined as a transient reduction in fetal heart rate of 15 beats per minute below the baseline, lasting for 15 seconds. In order to define a deceleration as late, early or variable, information is required regarding the timing of contractions. An acceleration on a CTG is defined as a transient increase in the fetal heart rate of 15 beats per minute lasting for more than 15 seconds. Two or more accelerations in a 30-minute CTG recording are a positive sign of fetal health. The CTG may be used in conjunction with ultrasound findings to produce a biophysical profile.

See Chapter 6, *Obstetrics by Ten Teachers*, 19th edition.

12 Ultrasound measurements

1 D   2 F   3 G   4 C

Pregnancies should ideally be dated by ultrasound between 10 and 14 weeks. The crown–rump length is the most accurate parameter up to 13+6/40; thereafter the head circumference is used up to 20/40. The ratio between the head circumference and abdominal circumference is useful in assessing whether growth is restricted asymmetrically, when the head circumference will be proportionally larger due to brain sparing. Infants of diabetic mothers are at risk of fetal macrosomia and hence increased abdominal circumference. There are several algorithms for estimating fetal weight, including a combination of HC/AC/FL/BPD.

See Chapter 6, *Obstetrics by Ten Teachers*, 19th edition.

13 Prenatal diagnosis

1 I   **2** B   **3** H   **4** F

Ventriculomegaly can be seen on ultrasound scanning, but does not fit any of the options given. Down's syndrome screening can be undertaken in several ways, but the National Screening Committee recommends the combination of ultrasound for nuchal translucency and blood tests for human chorionic gonadotrophin (hCG) and pregnancy-associated plasma protein A (PAPP-A). Diseases that are caused by clonal expansion of trinucleotide repeats include fragile X, Huntingdon's disease, myotonic dystrophy and Fredriech's ataxia. Klinefelter's syndrome is the result of an XXY karyotype and gives the listed phenotypic features.

See Chapter 7, *Obstetrics by Ten Teachers*, 19th edition.

14 Modes of prenatal testing

1 G   **2** E   **3** H   **4** I

The main advantage of CVS over amniocentesis is that it can be performed earlier in the pregnancy. Cordo-centesis is a relatively unusual procedure, but can be performed where a fetal blood sample is required, for example to determine platelet count in suspected alloimmune thrombocytopaenia. Fetal DNA is present in small amounts in the maternal plasma during pregnancy. If the *SRY* gene can be detected in maternal peripheral blood then the fetus is male and hence at risk of X-linked disorders. In order to detect single-gene defects in the fetus, a sample of fetal cells must be obtained, which can be achieved only by invasive methods. The maternal plasma does not carry sufficient DNA that can be differentiated from maternal-circulating DNA to enable single-gene testing.

See Chapter 7, *Obstetrics by Ten Teachers*, 19th edition.

15 Antepartum haemorrhage

1 A   **2** H   **3** G   **4** B

The most likely diagnosis for a twin pregnancy presenting with painless vaginal bleeding is a placenta praevia. A twin pregnancy increases the area of the placenta and hence increases the chances of it being low within the uterine cavity. Small post-coital bleeds from the cervix are common during pregnancy, as the cervix softens. Vaginal infections are common in pregnancy and often present with a bloody discharge. A large placental abruption is a life-threatening event and prompt steps in maternal resuscitation must be taken. An abruption is acutely dangerous for both mother and fetus, so it is critical that it is recognized as soon as possible.

See Chapter 8, *Obstetrics by Ten Teachers*, 19th edition.

16 Fetal malpresentations

1 D   **2** A   **3** G   **4** E

Breech presentation can be in an extended, flexed or footling position. Only in a footling breech does the foot present below the breech. A transverse lie is defined as a lie perpendicular to the maternal long axis. An oblique lie occurs when the angle of the fetal to the maternal axis is close to 45 degrees. When the fetal lie is unstable (i.e. the longitudinal axis of the baby relative to the mother still fluctuates at term) there is a risk of cord prolapse if the membranes rupture, hence women are routinely admitted to hospital at term. An external cephalic version can turn a breech to cephalic presentation, with success rates of around 50 per cent.

See Chapter 8, *Obstetrics by Ten Teachers*, 19th edition.

17 Thromboprophylaxis

1 B   **2** D   **3** G   **4** F

Thromboprophylaxis in pregnancy and the puerperium in the UK is usually based on the RCOG guidelines (2009). The woman in statement 1 has a metallic mitral valve replacement and should be on lifelong anticoagulation. This is usually achieved with warfarin, but may be switched to low molecular weight heparin in pregnancy. Statement 2 requires extended post-natal clexane as she has had a previous VTE event and may well have also been on antenatal thromboprophylaxis. Statement 3 has a single VTE risk factor (parity >3) and therefore needs only sensible precautions. Statement 4 has an additional risk factor in being aged >35 and therefore needs post-natal low molecular weight heparin.

See Chapter 8, *Obstetrics by Ten Teachers*, 19th edition.

18 Common problems of pregnancy

1 H   **2** L   **3** D   **4** A

Minor complications of pregnancy are extremely common. A sympathetic but practical response from health-care professionals can greatly improve a woman's experience of pregnancy. Symphysis pubis dysfunction is excruciatingly painful if severe, but can be managed by a physiotherapist. Gastro-oesophageal reflux is usually caused by a combination of hormonal and pressure effects from the growing uterus. Fainting usually occurs early in pregnancy when shifts in cardiovascular function are happening and may be managed as above. Constipation is common due to reduced gut motility, and iron supplementation may exacerbate this.

See Chapter 8, *Obstetrics by Ten Teachers*, 19th edition.

19 Twins and higher order multiple gestations

1 B   **2** J   **3** H   **4** D

The lambda sign is observed when two amniotic sacs arise from different chorionic plates, the T sign is seen when amniotic sacs arise from the same chorion and no inter-twin membrane is present in monochorionic monoamniotic twins. Monozygotic twin pregnancies carry a higher risk of death or disability in the co-twin than dizygotic twins. Monzygotic twins splitting at 4–8 days will share a placenta but be within separate amniotic sacs. Earlier splitting will result in separate placentae as well as separate amniotic sacs.

See Chapter 9, *Obstetrics by Ten Teachers*, 19th edition.

20 Management of multiple pregnancy

1 A   **2** F   **3** B   **4** I

Monozygotic twin pregnancies are at higher risk of growth abnormalities (e.g. twin-to-twin transfusion syndrome) in the third trimester and will therefore be scanned at fortnightly intervals. Dizygotic twins will usually be scanned every 4–6 weeks if the pregnancy is otherwise uncomplicated. Multi-fetal reduction is a difficult decision for patients, as it increases the risk of miscarriage before viability, but decreases the risk of preterm birth. It may be an unacceptable procedure to patients. Monoamniotic monochorionic twins are usually delivered at 32–34/40 by elective Caesarean section.

See Chapter 9, *Obstetrics by Ten Teachers*, 19th edition.

21 The clinical management of hypertension in pregnancy

1 G   **2** D   **3** K   **4** B

In statement 1, the most likely problem is pre-eclampsia, but this requires confirmation with urinary protein quantification. This patient needs to be admitted for further investigation and to monitor her blood pressure to consider treatment. In statement 2, a 31-year-old woman who has a blood pressure of 145/85 has chronic hypertension and so requires monitoring of blood pressure. Oedema is common in late pregnancy. In statement 3, a blood pressure of 150–170/100–119 with significant proteinuria signifies pre-eclampsia. A blood pressure in this range requires treatment with intravenous hypertensives. Intravenous magnesium sulphate will also be appropriate, but magnesium hydroxide is not a treatment for pre-eclampsia. The woman in statement 4 likely has gestational hypertension as in her previous pregnancy and should be started on oral antihypertensive therapy. Pre-eclampsia does not present with elevated blood pressure at 12/40.

See Chapter 10, *Obstetrics by Ten Teachers*, 19th edition.

22 Features of abnormal placentation

1 C   **2** A   **3** H   **4** F

In statement 1, a seizure in labour in a non-epileptic with a raised blood pressure is highly likely to represent eclampsia. In statement 2, a mildly elevated blood pressure with a high ALT makes HELLP syndrome the most likely diagnosis. A full blood count and film are urgently required. Sudden onset of severe abdominal pain and bleeding in late pregnancy as in the third woman in statement 3 should always raise the suspicion of placental abruption. This is more common in the context of pre-eclampsia, and this may be the cause of her elevated blood pressure. The patient in statement 4 has a mildly elevated blood pressure but no protein in the urine, which suggests the diagnosis of gestational hypertension.

See Chapter 10, *Obstetrics by Ten Teachers*, 19th edition.

23 Late miscarriage

1 G   **2** F   **3** A   **4** B

Abdominal discomfort and suprapubic pain as displayed in statement 1 are common problems presenting to obstetricians. The urine dip results suggest that this is a urinary tract infection, which should be treated with antibiotics. The ruptured membranes and pyrexia in statement 2 are suggestive of chorioamnionitis. This needs treatment with intravenous antibiotics and careful consideration regarding the continuation of the pregnancy. The bleeding and abdominal pain in statement 3 are suggestive of threatened miscarriage. In statement 4, cervical dilatation and funnelling at 20/40 are indicative of cervical incompetence. Insertion of a cervical cerclage may be an appropriate treatment.

See Chapter 11, *Obstetrics by Ten Teachers*, 19th edition.

24 Risk factors for preterm labour

1 K   **2** F   **3** C   **4** A

The main risk of preterm labour in multiple pregnancy is the increased intrauterine volume, which leads to over-distension. Intrauterine bleeding, such as a subchorionic haemorrhage, is irritant to the uterus and may contribute to episodes of abdominal pain and bleeding. Surgery such as appendicectomy is relatively safe in pregnancy, but does increase the risk of preterm labour. Smoking is the only modifiable risk factor in the list. Help and encouragement to stop smoking should be offered.

See Chapter 11, *Obstetrics by Ten Teachers*, 19th edition.

25 Diagnosis and management of preterm delivery

1 E	2 H	3 F	4 G

Nitrazine testing uses the alkaline pH of amniotic fluid to test for rupture of the membranes. There are many reasons for a false positive result, but it has a high negative predictive value. Tocolysis has no significant effect in prolonging pregnancy to term, but may allow critical extra hours or days to optimize care before delivery. Cervical cerclage is appropriate only in a small group of carefully selected patients. The results of emergency cerclage are generally poor. Amniocentesis can be used to obtain a sample of amniotic fluid for microscopy, culture and sensitivities. This is not commonly performed in the UK.

See Chapter 11, *Obstetrics by Ten Teachers*, 19th edition.

26 Drugs used in pregnancy

1 E	2 F	3 B	4 I

In statement 1, ursodeoxycholic acid is used in the symptomatic treatment of obstetric cholestasis. It chelates bile acids and reduces the itching sensation. In statement 2, magnesium sulphate has been shown to reduce the chances of the patient having a second eclamptic seizure. In statement 3, the ORACLE trial demonstrated that erythromycin is the appropriate choice of antibiotic for preterm pre-labour rupture of the membranes. A woman presenting with tiredness, glycosuria and a fasting blood glucose of 8.1 mmol/L, as in statement 4, has diabetes and may require insulin to control blood glucose.

See Chapter 12, *Obstetrics by Ten Teachers*, 19th edition.

27 Shortness of breath in pregnancy

1 C	2 D	3 H	4 G

Three to 12 per cent of pregnant women are affected by asthma, which may get better or worse during pregnancy. In cystic fibrosis, multiple medical problems, including diabetes, malabsorption and pulmonary hypertension, may complicate pregnancy. Pregnancy does not significantly shorten survival but requires close monitoring and careful management of any problems arising. Pulmonary hypertension in pregnancy is associated with a high risk of maternal death (30–50 per cent). Clear contraceptive advice is essential. Women with stenotic heart lesions have difficulty in increasing their cardiac output sufficiently to meet the demands of pregnancy and therefore many experience worsening symptoms and breathlessness.

See Chapter 12, *Obstetrics by Ten Teachers*, 19th edition.

28 Perinatal infection (1)

1 E	2 A	3 F	4 G

Listeria monocytogenes is a Gram-positive rod. It is an important cause of a wide spectrum of human diseases. Toxoplasmosis is a protozoan that can produce congenital or post-natal infections in humans. Congenital infections occur when non-immune mothers are infected with the protozoan and are of greater severity. Fifth disease is caused by parvovirus B19.

See Chapter 13, *Obstetrics by Ten Teachers*, 19th edition.

29 Perinatal infection (2)

1 A   2 D   3 E   4 G

HIV-positive women are often advised to have an elective Caesarean section to reduce the chance of vertical transmission, but a vaginal delivery is an option for women taking triple drug antiretroviral therapy who have a viral load <50 copies/ml at the time of delivery. Women who are co-infected with hepatitis C should be advised to have a Caesarean section as the vertical transmission rate is higher in co-infection. Ninety per cent of adults in the UK are immune to varicella zoster. Initial treatment of syphilis with parenteral penicillin provokes the Jarisch-Herxheimer reaction due to a release of pro-inflammatory cytokines. Congenital rubella infection rate is 80 per cent in infants whose mothers had symptomatic infection during the first 12 weeks of pregnancy. Mothers who are found to be non-immune on routine testing should therefore be vaccinated after pregnancy. Vaccination during pregnancy is contraindicated due to a theoretical risk of congenital rubella syndrome from the live attenuated vaccine.

See Chapter 13, *Obstetrics by Ten Teachers*, 19th edition.

30 Mechanism of labour

1 F   2 B   3 H   4 C

The mechanism of labour refers to the series of changes that occurs in the position and attitude of the fetus during its passage through the birth canal. The process involves engagement, descent, flexion, internal rotation, extension, restitution, external rotation, and delivery of the shoulders and fetal body. Engagement is said to have occurred when the widest part of the presenting part has passed successfully through the inlet.

See Chapter 14, *Obstetrics by Ten Teachers*, 19th edition.

31 Stages of labour

1 B   2 G   3 H   4 A

The third stage is the time from delivery of the fetus until delivery of the placenta and membranes. The time at which the third stage should be considered abnormal may be increased to 60 minutes if the woman has opted for a 'physiological' third stage. The process of effacement may begin during the weeks preceding the onset of labour, but will be complete by the end of the latent phase. The active second stage conventionally lasts no longer than 2 hours in a primiparous woman and no longer than 1 hour in a woman who has had a previous vaginal delivery. The duration of the latent phase is highly variable and may be prolonged, especially in primiparous women.

See Chapter 14, *Obstetrics by Ten Teachers*, 19th edition.

32 Interventions in the second stage

1 H   2 C   3 I   4 E

In statement 1, the pathological trace will mandate expedited delivery, assuming that delivery is not already imminent. A ventouse delivery would be contraindicated at <35/50. In statement 2, the presenting diameter in a brow presentation is the occipto-mental, measuring 13 cm. Vaginal delivery will not be possible and emergency Caesarean section should therefore be carried out as soon as the diagnosis is confirmed. The woman in statement 3 has been actively pushing for only 30 minutes and the fetal head is still high in the pelvic canal. The mechanism of labour dictates that as long at the head is well flexed, it should rotate on reaching the sloping gutter formed by the levator ani muscles. Provided that there are no other concerns with mother or fetus, this woman should be allowed to continue attempting to gain descent of the fetal head through normal maternal effort. In the scenario in statement 4, descent of the fetal head has occurred with maternal effort, but rotation still has not been achieved despite adequate time allowed. An attempt should therefore be made to rotate and deliver the baby vaginally. Significant maternal effort is required for successful rotation and delivery with the ventouse, and Kielland's forceps are therefore the instrument of choice if an experienced operator is available.

See Chapter 15, *Obstetrics by Ten Teachers*, 19th edition.

33 Complications of Caesarean section

1 H   **2** G   **3** I   **4** A

Ileus and bowel injury may be difficult to distinguish as both present with pain, bloating and failure to pass flatus post-operatively. Ileus, however, tends to present earlier and the patient will maintain their vital signs. A digital rectal examination and further imaging are mandatory if the condition does not resolve. Diaphragmatic irritation from blood and fluid remaining within the peritoneal cavity is common after Caesarean section. Shoulder tip pain is the classical presentation, but this must be carefully distinguished from chest pathology with a respiratory examination and oxygen saturations/heart rate. Pulmonary embolus is a leading cause of maternal death and careful attention must therefore be paid to thromboprophylaxis in the puerperium. Caesarean hysterectomy is an uncommon but life-saving procedure, carried out after 1 in 1000 deliveries. The most important risk factor is a previous uterine scar, particularly with an overlying placenta increasing the risk of placenta accreta.

See Chapter 15, *Obstetrics by Ten Teachers*, 19th edition.

34 Obstetric emergencies

1 C   **2** E   **3** D

The history of a sudden onset of occipital headaches with associated vomiting should raise the suspicion of subarachnoid haemorrhage. The associated loss of consciousness would point to the diagnosis of subarachnoid haemorrhage. Although migraine and hypercalcaemia could present with this history, they are not options available. The definitive diagnosis would be confirmed with brain imaging. The combination of hypertension and proteinuria combined with a collapse would be eclampsia until proven otherwise.

See Chapter 16, *Obstetrics by Ten Teachers*, 19th edition.

35 Choose the obstetric emergency that each woman is at highest risk of experiencing

1 I   **2** A   **3** G   **4** F

In statement 1, shoulder dystocia carries a significant risk of fetal hypoxia, death and trauma. Risk factors include elevated body mass index (BMI), maternal diabetes, prolonged second stage and instrumental delivery. In statement 2, cord prolapse has an incidence of 1:500 deliveries and can lead to fetal hypoxia or death if it results in prolonged compression on the cord. Risk factors include prematurity and abnormal lie, in the presence of ruptured membranes. In statement 3, uterine rupture is uncommon, but the main risk factor is previous Caesarean section. Induction of labour makes this complication more likely. In statement 4, uterine inversion is a rare complication in the third stage. It is usually caused by excessive traction on the umbilical cord prior to placental separation.

See Chapter 16, *Obstetrics by Ten Teachers*, 19th edition.

36 Postpartum pyrexia

1 H   **2** F   **3** C

The most likely diagnosis of an enlarged uterus and associated temperature is retained products of conception. The woman initially needs blood cultures and intravenous antibiotics. This should be followed by a surgical evacuation of the uterus. The differential diagnosis for a woman who presents after a Caesarean section with a temperature and abdominal pain is a wound infection, uterine infection or urinary tract infection. Caesarean section increases the risk of uterine infection and this is confirmed by the presence of an offensive discharge. This is unlikely to be retained products, as the uterine cavity is checked manually after a Caesarean section. A urinary tract infection would have dysuria and urine analysis would be abnormal. The differential diagnosis of a woman who presents with a temperature and chest signs is a chest infection, pneumonia or pulmonary embolism. The most likely diagnosis with purulent sputum is pneumonia, which should be treated with antibiotics.
See Chapter 17, *Obstetrics by Ten Teachers*, 19th edition.

37 Postpartum contraception

1 H   **2** B   **3** G   **4** A

Intrauterine contraceptive devices should be placed once the uterine cavity has involuted closer to its original size and shape. There is also an excess risk of perforation if placed in a soft, postpartum uterus. Lactional amenorrhoea provides some contraceptive effect if an exclusive breastfeeding regime is followed, but many women prefer to have an additional means of contraception. Laparoscopic clip sterilization has a lower failure rate than sterilization at the time of Caesarean section. The oral contraceptive pill should be avoided in the puerperium as it increases the already higher risk of venous thromboembolism and because it can have an adverse effect on breast milk.
See Chapter 17, *Obstetrics by Ten Teachers*, 19th edition.

38 Psychiatric disorders in pregnancy and the puerperium

1 E   **2** F   **3** H   **4** A

Puerperal psychosis affects approximately 1 in 1000 women. It presents rarely before the third postpartum day, but usually does so before 4 weeks. The onset is characteristically abrupt, with a rapidly changing clinical picture. The patient should be referred urgently to a psychiatrist and will require admission to a psychiatric unit. It is common for women in the first 24–48 hours to experience an elevation in mood, a feeling of excitement and some overactivity. This is termed the post-natal 'pinks'. Bipolar affective disorder is usually controlled with a combination of mood-stabilizing drugs (lithium), antidepressants and neuroleptics. Lithium carries a risk of causing cardiac defects if used in the first trimester.
See Chapter 18, *Obstetrics by Ten Teachers*, 19th edition.

39 Neonatology

1 G   **2** C   **3** I

Respiratory distress syndrome commences at or shortly after birth. A strong causal factor is lack of pulmonary surfactant and hence the incidence of respiratory distress syndrome highly correlated with gestational age.

Damage to the lowest roots of the brachial plexus (C8 and T1) is unusual but includes Klumpke's palsy due to instances of the arm remaining above the head during breech delivery. Milia represent retention cysts of the pilosebaceous follicles and disappear spontaneously over 1–2 months.

See Chapter 19, *Obstetrics by Ten Teachers*, 19th edition.

40 Neonatal care

| 1 E | 2 A | 3 B | 4 C | 5 D |

In statement 1, infants at <29/40 gestation and <48 hours of age require maximal-intensity intensive care. The infant in statement 2 will need regular blood sugar monitoring as she is at risk of developing hypoglycaemia. In statement 4, babies having frequent apnoea attacks require high-dependency care, with staff caring for one or two babies at a time. The female infant in statement 5 is herself not in need of extra care but should remain in hospital until full psychiatric assessment of her mother has been completed. The post-natal ward can provide this level of care.

See Chapter 19, *Obstetrics by Ten Teachers*, 19th edition.

41 Neonatal screening

| 1 E | 2 C | 3 A | 4 G |

Breech babies are at increased risk of developmental dysplasia of the hip and should undergo ultrasound to screen for this. Ultrasound should also be performed for all babies with a positive Ortolani–Barlow test or a positive family history. Phenylketonuria is a single-gene defect included on the Guthrie card, as is cystic fibrosis. Screening for neuroblastoma with urinary vanillylmandelic acid (VMA) measurement has been trialled in Canada but has not proved cost effective. Treatment for congenital hypothyroidism within the first 28 days significantly affects IQ later in life.

See Chapter 19, *Obstetrics by Ten Teachers*, 19th edition.

CHAPTER 2

MULTIPLE CHOICE QUESTIONS

QUESTIONS

Please answer true (T) or false (F) to the following statements.

Obstetric history taking and examination

1   Obstetric history:
a) It is recommended that women are seen on their own at least once during antenatal care.
b) A family history of pre-eclampsia should trigger increased antenatal surveillance.
c) During pregnancy 3 per cent of women use illicit drugs.
d) A history of sub-fertility is important even if the patient is currently pregnant.
e) A woman who has had a previous ectopic pregnancy should be offered an early pregnancy ultrasound scan (USS).

2   The following terms are appropriate:
a) Lie: cephalic.
b) Position: flexed.
c) Station: at the level of the spines.
d) Engagement: two-fifths.
e) Presenting part: shoulder.

3   Antenatal screening in the UK is offered for:
a) Down's syndrome.
b) Hepatitis C.
c) Rubella.
d) Cystic fibrosis.
e) Fetal anomalies.

Modern maternity care

4   Aspects of care reviewed by the Clinical Negligence Scheme for Trusts include:
a) Hand washing.
b) Newborn care.
c) Caesarean section rate.
d) Communication.
e) High-risk conditions.

Physiological changes in pregnancy

5   In normal pregnancy:
a) Blood pressure falls in the second trimester.
b) Plasma volume decreases throughout gestation.
c) There is a 50 per cent reduction in erythrocyte production.
d) 80 per cent of women have a transient diastolic murmur.
e) There is an increase in polymorphonuclear leukocytes.

6   Maternal effects on the physiology of the kidney include:
a) There is a 40 per cent increase in renal blood flow.
b) There is an increase in glomerular filtration rate (GFR).
c) The urea and creatinine are higher than in the non-pregnant state.
d) Glycosuria indicates likely development of diabetes.
e) The kidneys increase in size.

7   Gastrointestinal changes in pregnancy include:
a) Increased transit time.
b) Increased incidence of dental caries.
c) Decreased oesophageal sphincter tone.
d) Increased gastric acidity.
e) Decreased albumin production by the liver.

8   Metabolism in pregnancy:
a) Relative insulin resistance is normal in late gestation.
b) High-density lipoprotein (HDL) cholesterol is elevated in pregnancy.
c) Average gestational weight gain is 12.5 kg.
d) Calcium is less readily absorbed from the gut in pregnancy.
e) Total body water increases by about 3 L.

9   Skin changes during normal pregnancy include:
a) Hypopigmentation.
b) Increased bruising.
c) Straie gravidarum.
d) Increased hirsutism.
e) Decreased acne.

Normal fetal development and growth

10   The following factors influence fetal birthweight:
a) The parity of the mother.
b) The exercise habits of the mother.
c) The ethnicity of the mother.

d) The sex of the fetus.

e) Maternal folate supplementation.

11 During lung development:

a) Surfactant production occurs from about 20 weeks.

b) The predominant phospholipid is phosphatidylcholine.

c) The majority of infants born at 27/40 experience some degree of respiratory distress syndrome.

d) Fetal breathing movement occurs least during REM sleep.

e) The production of lecithin is enhanced by cortisol and diabetes.

12 Regarding the fetal liver:

a) Glycogen is stored in large quantities in the third trimester.

b) The enzymes required to conjugate bilirubin are not present.

c) Red blood cell manufacture begins at 20/40.

d) Derives from the mesoderm.

e) Has the same embryological origin as the gall bladder.

Antenatal care

13 With regard to routine antenatal care:

a) All women should be offered screening for haemoglobinopathies.

b) A high vaginal swab should be sent routinely at booking.

c) Syphilis testing forms part of the routine booking visit.

d) An ultrasound scan for anomalies should be performed at 24/40.

e) Every patient should have a named consultant.

Antenatal imaging and assessment of fetal well-being

14 Considering Doppler ultrasound:

a) Abnormal uterine artery Doppler flow indicates fetal hypoxaemia.

b) Abnormal umbilical artery flow indicates poor placental perfusion.

c) Fetal hypoxaemia is associated with redistribution of blood flow.

d) Fetal anaemia is best assessed using measurements from the middle cerebral artery.

e) Abnormal ductus venosus blood flow occurs prior to arterial changes.

15 The following are evaluated when performing a fetal biophysical profile:

a) Estimated fetal weight.

b) Fetal tone.

c) Maternal blood pressure.

d) Amniotic fluid volume.

e) Placental blood flow.

16 The aims of the 18–22 weeks anomaly scan include:

a) To locate the placenta.

b) To determine the chorionicity of a twin pregnancy.

c) Assessment of amniotic fluid volume.

d) Promoting parental bonding with the fetus.

e) To identify fetal structural defects.

Prenatal diagnosis

17 The following statements are true for prenatal tests:

a) Serum biochemistry is superior to maternal age as a screening test for Down's syndrome.

b) Maternal serum alpha-fetoprotein is a diagnostic test for neural tube defects.
c) Amniocentesis has a higher pregnancy loss rate than chorionic villus sampling.
d) Tests using DNA technology can be performed on amniocentesis specimens.
e) Chorionic villus sampling can be performed only before 12 weeks' gestation.

18 Considering neural tube defects:
a) These occur as a result of a poor peri-conceptual maternal diet.
b) The majority of these defects occur at the end of the spine.
c) The prognosis for spina bifida depends on the level of the lesion.
d) With a previous affected sibling the risk of recurrence is 1 per cent.
e) A supplement of 5 mg folic acid significantly reduces the risk of recurrence.

19 Chorionic villus sampling:
a) Carries a 2 per cent risk of causing miscarriage.
b) May show a placental mosaic phenotype.
c) May be unsuccessful in obtaining a sample.
d) The most common approach is transcervical.
e) May be carried out at <11/40.

Antenatal obstetric complications

20 Oligohydramnios is associated with the following:
a) Tracheo-oesophageal fistula.
b) Talipes.
c) Intrauterine growth restriction.
d) Anencephaly.
e) Premature rupture of the fetal membranes.

21 Polyhydramnios is associated with the following:
a) Maternal diabetes.
b) Neuromuscular fetal conditions.
c) Maternal non-steroidal anti-inflammatory drugs (NSAIDs).
d) Post-maturity.
e) Chorioangioma of the placenta.

22 During an assisted breech delivery:
a) An episiotomy may be cut once the anus is seen at the fourchette.
b) Pinard's manoeuvre can be used to deliver the legs in an extended position.
c) Mauriceau–Smellie–Veit is used to deliver extended arms.
d) Forceps should not be applied to the fetal head.
e) Epidural analgesia is mandatory.

23 The following are contraindications to external cephalic version:
a) Polyhydramnios.
b) Complete breech position.
c) Pre-eclampsia.
d) Symphysis pubis dysfunction.
e) Twin pregnancy.

Twins and higher multiple gestations

24 In vaginal twin delivery:
a) The first twin is at greater risk than the second.
b) The second twin must be delivered within 15 minutes of the first.
c) Labour usually occurs prior to term.
d) Internal podalic version is a useful strategy for delivery of the first twin.
e) There is an increased risk of postpartum haemorrhage.

25 Monozygotic twins:
a) Always have a risk of cord entanglement.
b) Each twin has a risk of structural abnormality four times higher than a single fetus.
c) If diamniotic, they are separated by a membrane carrying the lambda sign.
d) If monochorionic, twins have a 15 per cent chance of developing twin-to-twin transfusion syndrome (TTTS).
e) Cannot be dichorionic diamniotic.

26 Higher-order multiple pregnancies:
a) Replacement of only two embryos in *in vitro* fertilization (IVF) protocols prevents the risk of triplet pregnancy.
b) The median gestational age of delivery of triplets is 33/40.
c) Evidence strongly suggests that triplets should be delivered by elective Caesarean section.
d) If opting for multi-fetal reduction, this should be carried out as soon after diagnosis as possible.
e) Multi-fetal reduction increases the chance of pregnancy loss before viability.

Pre-eclampsia and other disorders of placentation

27 With regard to the placenta:
a) It receives the highest blood flow of any fetal organ.
b) The resistance of the spiral arterioles increases significantly in the second trimester.
c) Abnormally increased bore of the spiral arteries contributes to pathogenesis in pre-eclampsia.
d) It is a major endocrine organ.
e) Each cotelydon contains a primary stem villus.

28 Pre-eclampsia is more common in:
a) Multigravid women.
b) Women with congenital cardiac disease.
c) Multiple pregnancy.
d) Women with diabetes insipidus.
e) Women with pre-existing renal disease.

29 The management of pre-eclampsia includes:
a) Hospital assessment.
b) Labetalol.
c) Early delivery.
d) Frusemide.
e) Magnesium sulphate.

30 The following are risk factors for intrauterine growth restriction:
a) Multiple pregnancy.
b) Aspirin use in pregnancy.
c) Antiphospholipid syndrome.
d) Fetal karyotype anomalies.
e) Maternal age >35.

31 Consequences of placental abruption include:
a) Hypovolaemic shock.
b) Fetal anaemia.
c) Amniotic fluid embolus.
d) Increased perinatal mortality.
e) Intrauterine death.

Late miscarriage and early birth

32 Second trimester miscarriage:
a) Is typically painless.
b) Occurs between 12 and 24 weeks' gestation.
c) Can be associated with rupture of the fetal membranes.
d) May be associated with haemorrhage, infection and multiple pregnancy.
e) Antibiotic prophylaxis is usually given.

33 In evaluating a patient with suspected pre-labour rupture of the membranes:
a) Maternal baseline blood tests should be performed.
b) A digital examination to assess cervical dilatation should be performed.
c) A transabdominal ultrasound scan may help decide whether the membranes have ruptured.
d) A speculum examination is best performed immediately after the patient has mobilized to empty the bladder.
e) A fetal cardiotocograph should always be performed.

34 Antenatal steroid administration:
a) Is indicated in threatened preterm labour from 24/40 until 37/40.
b) Is of no benefit if delivery does not occur within 1 week of administration.
c) Should not be performed unless the diagnosis of preterm labour is confirmed.
d) Has not been shown to cause developmental problems following single doses.
e) Tocolysis may be indicated to allow steroids to take effect.

35 The following drugs have been shown to be effective in the treatment of preterm labour:
a) Atosiban.
b) Pethidine.
c) Nifedipine.
d) Labetalol.
e) Ritodrine.

36 The risks of premature preterm rupture of the fetal membranes include:
a) Premature labour.
b) Cord prolapse.
c) Pre-eclampsia.

d) Maternal septicaemia.

e) Antepartum haemorrhage.

Medical diseases complicating pregnancy

37 Patients diagnosed as having mitral stenosis:

a) Usually have been diagnosed prior to pregnancy.

b) Should not take beta-blockers during pregnancy.

c) Should not have diuretic therapy during pregnancy.

d) Could be considered for mitral valvotomy during pregnancy.

e) Have a risk of adverse fetal outcome related to the severity of the mitral stenosis.

38 Considering cystic fibrosis in pregnancy:

a) The partner does not need genetic testing.

b) This is an autosomal recessive disorder.

c) The woman should have an oral glucose tolerance test.

d) Caesarean section is mandatory owing to poor lung function.

e) Fetal growth should be monitored with serial ultrasound scanning.

39 With reference to iron deficiency anaemia in pregnancy:

a) Iron demand in pregnancy increases to 4 mg per day.

b) High levels of serum ferritin confirm the diagnosis.

c) It is more common in multiple pregnancy.

d) It is usually treated with oral iron.

e) Blood transfusion should be avoided.

40 In relation to women who embark on pregnancy with a diagnosis of epilepsy:

a) Carbamazepine is associated with neural tube defects.

b) Breastfeeding is contraindicated in mothers taking anticonvulsants.

c) Vitamin K should be commenced from 30 weeks' gestation.

d) Women on multiple drug therapy should be changed to monotherapy if possible.

e) Intravenous magnesium sulphate is the best management of status epilepticus in labour.

Perinatal infections

41 With regard to congenital infection with cytomegalovirus:

a) It is characterized by intracerebral calcification.

b) It is a recognized cause of microcephaly.

c) It can be detected by culture of the infant's urine.

d) It is a cause of developmental delay.

e) 90 per cent of infections are asymptomatic.

42 Congenital malformation can be attributed to maternal infection with:

a) Poliomyelitis.

b) Toxoplasmosis.

c) Varicella zoster.

d) Parvovirus.

e) Syphilis.

43 Considering human immunodeficiency virus (HIV):
a) It is a retrovirus.
b) The antibody test may take one month to become positive after exposure.
c) There is no contraindication to fetal blood sampling if required in labour.
d) Advising against breastfeeding is an effective way of reducing vertical transmission.
e) With intervention the vertical transmission rate can be reduced to about 3 per cent.

Labour

44 With regard to the anatomy of the maternal pelvis:
a) The pudendal nerve passes in front of the ischial spine.
b) The anterior–posterior (AP) diameter of the pelvic inlet is 11 cm.
c) The anterior–posterior diameter of the pelvic outlet is 11 cm.
d) The levator ani muscles form the pelvic floor.
e) The angle of the inlet to the horizontal can be up to 90°.

45 Considering the fetal skull:
a) The anterior fontanelle is diamond shaped.
b) The sutures of the vault are ossified.
c) The vertex presentation longitudinal diameter is sub-occipito-frontal diameter.
d) The occipito-mental diameter is normally too large to pass through the maternal pelvis.
e) Moulding of the fetal skull is a normal physiological process.

46 Progress in labour is measured by:
a) The frequency of uterine contractions.
b) The force of uterine contractions.
c) Descent of the presenting part.
d) Dilatation of the cervix.
e) The length of time since rupture of the membranes.

47 In relation to the mechanism of labour:
a) Engagement is said to have occurred when the widest part of the fetal head has passed through the false pelvis.
b) Restitution occurs after external rotation.
c) Extension occurs after internal rotation.
d) Extension occurs at 'crowning'.
e) Descent of the fetal head is needed before flexion internal rotation and extension can occur.

48 Regarding face presentation:
a) This occurs in 1:50 labours.
b) The presenting diameter is submento-bregmatic, which is 9.5 cm.
c) It is commonly due to fetal thyroid tumours.
d) The face can deliver vaginally with the chin mento-anterior.
e) Oxytocin should be used to augment slow progress.

49 Considering the Bishop score:
a) It includes the station of the presenting part.
b) It includes the length of the cervical canal.
c) It includes the gestation of the fetus.

d) It includes the parity of the mother.

e) A score of 4 indicates that the cervix is unfavourable.

50 Concerning brow presentation:

a) The eyes, nose and mouth will be palpable vaginally.

b) It is the least common malposition.

c) The presenting diameter is mento-vertical.

d) It may be treated in labour by Caesarean section.

e) This is incompatible with vaginal delivery.

51 Vaginal bleeding in the first stage of labour may be due to:

a) Placental abruption.

b) Cervical fibroids.

c) Ruptured uterus.

d) Vaginal trauma.

e) Vasa praevia.

Operative intervention in obstetrics

52 Kielland's forceps:

a) Have a pelvic curvature.

b) Have a cephalic curvature.

c) Have a sliding lock.

d) Are used to rotate to an occipito-posterior position.

e) Should not be used under pudendal block analgesia alone.

Obstetric emergencies

53 With regard to shoulder dystocia:

a) It occurs in approximately 1 per cent of labours.

b) It is more common in assisted vaginal delivery.

c) McRobert's manoeuvre will be effective in 90 per cent of cases.

d) Fundal pressure should be avoided.

e) Avoid lateral flexion of the head on the neck.

54 The symptoms of pre-eclampsia include:

a) Restlessness.

b) Sleepiness.

c) Flashing lights in vision.

d) Rash.

e) Epigastric pain.

55 Initial management of severe postpartum haemorrhage requires:

a) Facial oxygen.

b) Administration of IV fluids via a central line.

c) Senior haematologist present.

d) Senior anaesthetist present.

e) Ultrasound scan of the uterus.

56 Extra factors to consider in maternal resuscitation include:
a) Tilting of the gravid abdomen.
b) Large breasts creating difficulties in ventilation.
c) Need for perimortem Caesarean section.
d) Increased functional lung capacity.
e) Lower risk of aspiration.

The puerperium

57 Human milk has the following advantages over formula milk:
a) Human milk contains more protein.
b) Human milk contains more lactose.
c) Human milk is associated with a reduction in atopic illness.
d) Human milk contains more iron.
e) Human milk is a good source of vitamin K.

58 The following are risk factors for puerperal infection:
a) Prolonged rupture of the membranes.
b) Prolonged pregnancy.
c) Prolonged second stage.
d) Caesarean section.
e) Home birth.

59 The following complications are more common after instrumental delivery:
a) Anaemia.
b) Prolonged perineal discomfort.
c) Mastitis.
d) Obstetric palsy.
e) Puerperal infection.

Psychiatric disorders and the puerperium

60 Post-natal blues:
a) Usually start between days 3 and 5.
b) May be prolonged by anaemia.
c) Are more common in women who have had normal deliveries.
d) Are prevented by night sedation.
e) Occur mostly in women who are discharged early from hospital.

61 Screening for mental illness during pregnancy:
a) Every woman should have a mental health history recorded at booking.
b) Women established on psychotropic drug therapy should cease their medication as soon as pregnancy is confirmed.
c) All women should be screened for depression at least twice in the post-natal period.
d) A family history of mental health problems is unlikely to be relevant.
e) If inpatient care is required post-natally, it is better that the baby should be cared for elsewhere.

Neonatology

62 Neonatal jaundice is a recognized feature of:
a) ABO incompatibility.
b) Glucose-6-phosphate dehydrogenase.

c) Rhesus incompatibility.
d) Ebstein's anomaly.
e) Meninigitis.

63 In haemorrhagic disease of the newborn:
a) Vitamin K prophylaxis is offered at birth to babies at high risk of haemorrhagic disease of the newborn.
b) A single oral dose of vitamin K is less effective than an intramuscular dose at preventing late-onset vitamin K deficiency bleeding.
c) Haemorrhagic disease of the newborn is treated with fresh frozen plasma.
d) Classical vitamin K deficiency bleeding presents within the first 48 hours.
e) Late-onset vitamin K deficiency bleeding is usually seen in babies whose mothers were on medication such as warfarin and anticonvulsants.

64 For neonatal resuscitation:
a) Ratio of chest compressions to breaths should be 15:2.
b) Five inflation breaths should be given initially, each lasting 1–2 seconds.
c) Naxolone should be considered if the mother has recently been given pethidine.
d) Chest compressions should be at a rate of 60 beats per minute.
e) If a baby looks pale during resuscitation, a blood transfusion should be considered.

Ethical and medicolegal issues in obstetric practice

65 Informed consent requires that a patient should:
a) Be able to understand the benefits of the proposed treatment.
b) Sign a formal written consent form.
c) Understand the consequences of refusing the proposed treatment.
d) Be able to retain and weigh up the information provided.
e) Be given several hours to consider and evaluate the options.

MCQ ANSWERS

1 T, T, F, T, T

Seeing women alone during antenatal care may encourage disclosure of domestic violence or other social problems. Approximately 0.5–1 per cent of women use illicit drugs during pregnancy, and this should trigger increased fetal monitoring and social support. A history of sub-fertility requiring assisted conception techniques is relevant to care later in the pregnancy. The rate of preterm delivery is higher in assisted conceptions and pre-eclampsia is more common with donated gametes. Women who have previously experienced ectopic pregnancy should have an early scan to confirm an intrauterine pregnancy.
See Chapter 1, *Obstetrics by Ten Teachers*, 19th edition.

2 F, F, T, T, T

The fetal lie can be longitudinal, transverse or oblique depending on the position of the fetal axis relative to the maternal axis. Engagement is described in terms of fifths of the fetal head palpable above the pubic symphysis. Station is described in terms of centimetres above or below the ischial spines. Fetuses in a transverse lie often present with the shoulder.
See Chapter 1, *Obstetrics by Ten Teachers*, 19th edition.

3 T, F, T, F, T

Antenatal screening is not routinely offered for hepatitis C, as there are no available interventions in the event of a positive result. Cystic fibrosis can be diagnosed on invasive fetal testing if there is a specific indication (both parents test positive as carriers), but is not routinely screened for in the antenatal period.
See Chapter 1, *Obstetrics by Ten Teachers*, 19th edition.

4 F, T, F, T, T

The Clinical Negligence Scheme for Trusts evaluates organization, clinical care, high-risk conditions, communications and newborn care.
See Chapter 2, *Obstetrics by Ten Teachers*, 19th edition.

5 T, F, F, F, T

Profound changes occur in the cardiovascular system during normal pregnancy. Blood pressure falls in the second trimester and then increases again in the third. Plasma volume is increased by about 50 per cent during gestation. This leads to a drop in haematocrit, despite an increase in total haemoglobin and erythrocyte production. A transient systolic murmur occurs frequently in pregnancy, but a diastolic murmur should raise the suspicion of pathology.
See Chapter 3, *Obstetrics by Ten Teachers*, 19th edition.

6 F, T, F, F, T

Renal blood flow increases by about 80 per cent in the second trimester, accompanied by an increase in glomerular filtration rate. Dilutional effects and increased GFR account for the fall in urea and creatinine. It is common in late pregnancy for glucose to spill over into the urine, and diabetes should be diagnosed on formal glucose tolerance testing. Mild hydronephrosis is common during pregnancy. It is more common in the right kidney due to extrinsic compression from the dextrorotated uterus.
See Chapter 3, *Obstetrics by Ten Teachers*, 19th edition.

7 T, T, T, T, F

Transit time increases during pregnancy because of the relaxant effect of progesterone on smooth muscle. The same effect accounts for decreased oesophageal sphincter tone. Albumin measured in the plasma is decreased during pregnancy, but this reflects a dilutional effect despite increased production by the liver.

See Chapter 3, *Obstetrics by Ten Teachers*, 19th edition.

8 T, T, T, F, F

Weight gain during pregnancy includes products of conception, increase in maternal tissues and increase in fat stores. Total weight gain is usually around 12.5 kg, and total body water increases by about 8 L. Calcium gut absorption is increased during pregnancy as a result of increased production of a vitamin D metabolite. HDL cholesterol increases by 12/40 and remains high during gestation.

See Chapter 3, *Obstetrics by Ten Teachers*, 19th edition.

9 F, F, T, T, F

Hyperpigmentation affects almost 90 per cent of pregnant women. This is reflected in darkening of the linea alba to the linea nigra. Acne tends to increase during pregnancy due to over-activity of the sebaceous glands. Increased hirsutism is common, and scalp hair may become thicker due to a prolonged anagen phase.

See Chapter 3, *Obstetrics by Ten Teachers*, 19th edition.

10 T, F, T, T, F

Fetal birthweight is influenced by a multitude of factors. Increased parity is associated with increased birthweight. Gentle exercise during pregnancy has not been demonstrated to reduce fetal birthweight. Certain ethnic groups tend to have smaller or larger babies, and male fetuses are generally larger than females. Maternal folate supplementation is important to prevent neural tube defects but does not directly influence birthweight.

See Chapter 4, *Obstetrics by Ten Teachers*, 19th edition.

11 F, T, T, F, F

Type I and II epithelial cells begin to differentiate at around 26/40 and surfactant production occurs from around 30/40. Phosphatidylcholine (lecithin) accounts for around 80 per cent of the phospholipid produced by type II pneumocytes. >80 per cent of infants born 23–27/40 will experience respiratory distress syndrome. Fetal breathing movement is frequent during rapid eye movement (REM) sleep. The production of lecithin is increased by cortisol and other factors that stress the fetus. Diabetes delays lecithin production and leaves the infant of the diabetic mother at higher risk of respiratory distress syndrome.

See Chapter 4, *Obstetrics by Ten Teachers*, 19th edition.

12 T, T, F, F, T

Glycogen laid down in the liver is important in protecting against neonatal hypoglycaemia. The enzymes that conjugate bilirubin are induced in the fetal liver after birth. Antenatally, bilirubin is transported via the placenta. The liver begins haematopoesis by week 6. The liver, pancreas and gall bladder are all out-pouchings of the endoderm that forms the fetal gut.

See Chapter 4, *Obstetrics by Ten Teachers*, 19th edition.

13 T, F, T, F, F

Pelvic examination does not form part of routine antenatal care. A vaginal swab may be sent if pelvic examination is indicated for another reason. Syphilis testing is part of routine screening bloods along with rubella, hepatitis B and HIV. The anomaly scan is performed at 18–22/40. Women with high-risk pregnancies should be booked under a named consultant. Low-risk women are suitable for midwifery-led care.

See Chapter 5, *Obstetrics by Ten Teachers*, 19th edition.

14 F, T, T, T, F

Abnormal uterine artery Doppler indices are used as indicators for an increased risk of pre-eclampsia and intrauterine growth restriction. Fetal anaemia is associated with a hyperdynamic circulation, whereas fetal hypoxaemia is associated with redistribution of blood flow. Abnormal flow in the ductus venosus is a pre-terminal observation and does not precede arterial changes.

See Chapter 6, *Obstetrics by Ten Teachers*, 19th edition.

15 F, T, F, T, F

Fetal biophysical profile involves assessment of a CTG tracing plus ultrasound assessment of fetal breathing movements, fetal body movements, fetal tone and amniotic fluid volume.

See Chapter 6, *Obstetrics by Ten Teachers*, 19th edition.

16 T, F, T, F, T

At the 18–22/40 anomaly scan, women with a low-lying placenta can be identified and followed up with a further scan to determine a group of women in whom the placenta will remain low-lying. The chorionicity of the pregnancy is best determined at the dating scan at 12/40. Fetal structural defects are generally apparent at 18–22/40 as morphogenesis is mostly complete.

See Chapter 6, *Obstetrics by Ten Teachers*, 19th edition.

17 T, F, F, T, F

Serum biochemistry has a sensitivity of 60–70 per cent, compared with 30–40 per cent for maternal age alone. The measurement of serum alpha-fetoprotein is a screening test for neural tube defects rather than a diagnostic test. Chorionic villus sampling has a higher rate of pregnancy loss than amniocentesis, although both are low in experienced hands. Either technique will involve obtaining fetally derived cells on which DNA testing can be performed.

See Chapter 7, *Obstetrics by Ten Teachers*, 19th edition.

18 F, T, T, F, T

Neural tube defects are among the most common major abnormalities. The aetiology is multi-factorial, with well-defined environmental, genetic, pharmacological and geographical factors implicated. Around 70–80 per cent of neural tube defects are anencephaly or encephaloceles. When a parent or previous sibling has had an NTD, the risk of recurrence is 5–10 per cent. Pre-conceptual folate supplementation of the maternal diet reduces the risk of developing these defects by about half. The dose of folic acid is 400 micrograms for primary prevention and 5 milligrams for women wishing to prevent a recurrence of an NTD.

See Chapter 7, *Obstetrics by Ten Teachers*, 19th edition.

19 T, T, T, F, F

The risk of causing miscarriage from chorionic villus sampling is usually quoted as 2 per cent, although it may be less in experienced hands. It is possible to perform CVS without obtaining a usable sample and the patient must be warned of this outcome in advance. CVS may be performed transvaginally, but the trans-abdominal route is more common. The earliest gestation at which CVS is recommended is 11/40.

See Chapter 7, *Obstetrics by Ten Teachers*, 19th edition.

20 F, T, T, F, T

A tracheo-oesophageal fistula causes polyhydramnios by preventing the normal mechanism of fetal swallowing. Anencephaly also causes severe polyhydramnios by preventing fetal swallowing. Talipes is associated with oligohydramnios due to the decreased intrauterine space. Intrauterine growth restriction is associated with oligohydramnios that is usually not as severe as that caused by fetal anomalies. Premature rupture of the membranes causes oligohydramnios via fluid loss.

See Chapter 8, *Obstetrics by Ten Teachers*, 19th edition.

21 T, T, F, F, T

Maternal diabetes associated with polyhydramnios needs urgent intervention as it often indicates high glucose levels. Fetal neuromuscular conditions interfere with swallowing and therefore are associated with polyhydramnios. Maternal NSAIDs reduce fetal renal function and hence slow the production of liquor. Cessation of NSAID use may allow reaccumulation of amniotic fluid. Chorioangioma of the placenta is associated with increased amniotic fluid volume.

See Chapter 8, *Obstetrics by Ten Teachers*, 19th edition.

22 T, T, F, F, F

An episiotomy should not be cut before the anterior buttock has been delivered and the anus is visible. Pinard's manoeuvre is used to flex the legs at the knee and hence safely deliver the extended legs. Mauriceau Smellie Veit manoeuvre is used to deliver the after-coming fetal head. Piper's forceps may be useful in delivering the fetal head. Epidural analgesia may be useful in any delivery that is expected to require vaginal manipulation or has a high chance of being converted to emergency Caesarean section, but is never mandatory for the patient.

See Chapter 8, *Obstetrics by Ten Teachers*, 19th edition.

23 T, F, T, F, T

External cephalic version is a straightforward technique with a low risk of adverse events that can reduce the requirement for elective Caesarean section in breech presentations. It is not performed in cases where there is concern about the well-being of the fetus such as polyhydramnios or pre-eclampsia, or where it is unlikely to be successful such as twin pregnancy or uterine abnormalities. Intrapartum external cephalic version may be performed after delivery of the first twin to deliver the second twin, but should not be performed antenatally.

See Chapter 8, *Obstetrics by Ten Teachers*, 19th edition.

24 F, F, T, F, T

Twin pregnancies account for 1.5 per cent of pregnancies in the UK. Intrapartum complications are more common with the second twin than with the first. Provided there are no concerns with the CTG of the second twin, there is no absolute interval length that must be achieved between the delivery of twins; however, the majority are delivered within 15 minutes. Spontaneous preterm labour is always a risk in twin pregnancy, where the average gestation is 37 rather than 40 weeks. Internal podalic version may be a useful strategy for delivery of the second twin, but would be inappropriate for the first. The increased distension of the uterus during twin pregnancy gives a greater likelihood of postpartum haemorrhage and a prophylactic syntocinon infusion is usually given postpartum.

See Chapter 9, *Obstetrics by Ten Teachers*, 19th edition.

25 F, T, F, T, F

Monozygotic twins within separate amniotic sacs (diamniotic) cannot get entangled within each other's cords. However, this risk is high approaching term with monoamniotic monochorionic twins. Monzygotic twins may be either di- or monochorionic, depending on when splitting of the conceptus occurs. If they are diamniotic they could therefore display either the T or lambda sign. Monochorionic twins have a 15 per cent chance of developing twin-to-twin transfusion syndrome and should be followed with repeated growth scans in the third trimester.

See Chapter 9, *Obstetrics by Ten Teachers*, 19th edition.

26 F, T, F, F, T

Assisted conception contributes to the increased risk of triplet pregnancy over the baseline population rate in the UK. IVF protocols are usually limited to replacing one or two embryos, but this does not prevent the relatively common occurrence of splitting of one embryo to give triplets composed of a monozygotic twin pair and a singleton. Triplets are usually delivered by elective Caesarean section in the UK, but limited available evidence suggests that vaginal birth gives comparable neonatal outcomes. Multi-fetal reduction should be carried out around 11–12 weeks to account for natural pregnancy loss. Although it reduces the chances of severe preterm birth, multi-fetal reduction increases the chance of pregnancy loss before viability.
See Chapter 9, *Obstetrics by Ten Teachers*, 19th edition.

27 T, F, F, T, T

The placenta receives the highest blood flow of any fetal organ, and by term the blood flow per minute is as high as 500–750 ml. In normal pregnancy, the effect of invasion of the trophoblast into the spiral arterioles is to convert them into large-bore, low-resistance, large-capacitance vessels. This creates a low-resistance shunt to supply the fetoplacental unit. Failure of this process is thought to contribute to the mechanism of pre-eclampsia and IUGR. The placenta is responsible for production of several hormones during pregnancy, including human placental lactogen. The placenta is divided into cotyledons, each of which contains a primary stem villus.
See Chapter 10, *Obstetrics by Ten Teachers*, 19th edition.

28 F, F, T, F, T

Pre-eclampsia is more common in primigravid women, women with diabetes mellitus (not diabetes insipidus) and women with pre-existing renal disease. Multiple pregnancy is also a risk factor, possibly linked to the greater placental area.
See Chapter 10, *Obstetrics by Ten Teachers*, 19th edition.

29 T, T, T, F, T

Hospital assessment is advised in pre-eclampsia to allow the severity of the condition to be quantified via continuous assessment of the blood pressure and serial haematological and biochemical parameters. Delivery will cure the condition. Labetalol is useful in lowering maternal blood pressure, and magnesium sulphate is used primarily for seizure prophylaxis. Frusemide is not helpful in the treatment of pre-eclampsia, as intravascular volume is usually depleted.
See Chapter 10, *Obstetrics by Ten Teachers*, 19th edition.

30 T, F, T, T, F

The higher total demand on the oxygen and glucose that can be supplied via the placenta means that fetuses in multiple pregnancies are often relatively growth restricted. Aspirin is commonly prescribed to pregnant women at increased risk of micro- or macrovascular thrombosis, and does not confer increased risk of IUGR. Antiphospholipid syndrome and fetal karyotype abnormalities are both risk factors. Advanced maternal age may confer an increased risk of pre-eclampsia or other conditions, but is not an independent risk factor for IUGR.
See Chapter 10, *Obstetrics by Ten Teachers*, 19th edition.

31 T, F, F, T, T

Placental abruption results in blood loss from the maternal circulation rather than the fetal. Hence hypo volaemic shock in the mother is common, but fetal anaemia is not. Increased perinatal mortality and intra uterine death are as a consequence of reduced placental perfusion and fetal hypoxia, rather than fetal blood loss. Amniotic fluid embolism is not associated with abruption.
See Chapter 10, *Obstetrics by Ten Teachers*, 19th edition.

32 F, T, T, T, F

Second trimester miscarriage typically presents with backache, contractions and vaginal bleeding. Rupture of the fetal membranes can be a feature. Antibiotics are given if there is evidence of infection.
See Chapter 11, *Obstetrics by Ten Teachers*, 19th edition.

33 T, F, T, F, F

Infection is a major concern in pre-labour rupture of the membranes. The cervix should be evaluated with a sterile speculum examination rather than a digital examination to reduce the risk of introducing infection. This should ideally be performed after the mother has been supine for some time to help identify amniotic fluid pooling in the speculum. A fetal CTG is useful in late gestation, but this is not helpful if the membranes rupture before the time of viability.
See Chapter 11, *Obstetrics by Ten Teachers*, 19th edition.

34 F, F, F, T, T

Steroids are not generally considered to be useful beyond 34 weeks, as the incidence of respiratory distress syndrome is down to 5 per cent at 35/40. Courses received less than 48 hours or more than 7 days from delivery are still of benefit. Antenatal steroids can be given on the suspicion of preterm labour, but care should be taken with multiple doses. There is no evidence of adverse effects after single doses. Tocolysis does not significantly prolong pregnancy, but may give critical extra time for steroid administration or *in utero* transfer.
See Chapter 11, *Obstetrics by Ten Teachers*, 19th edition.

35 T, F, T, F, T

Ritodrine is sympathomimetic and causes uterine relaxation. Nifedipine can be used to arrest preterm delivery as it acts to inhibit intracellular calcium release. Atosiban is a specific oxytocin receptor antagonist and therefore reduces uterine contractions. Labetalol is an alpha- and beta-receptor antagonist used in the reduction of blood pressure. Pethidine sedates the mother and the fetus but does not affect contractions.
See Chapter 11, *Obstetrics by Ten Teachers*, 19th edition.

36 T, T, F, T, F

The risks of premature rupture of the membranes include premature labour, malpresentation, cord prolapse and infection. Any woman delivering after preterm rupture of the fetal membranes is at risk of postpartum haemorrhage and endometritis.
See Chapter 11, *Obstetrics by Ten Teachers*, 19th edition.

37 T, F, F, T, T

The most common cause of mitral stenosis is rheumatic fever and it is therefore relatively uncommon in pregnant women in the UK. The problems with mitral stenosis in pregnancy stem from the inability of the stenotic valve to cope with the increase in cardiac output that pregnancy demands. Beta-blockers and diuretics may both be helpful in off-setting this demand. Mitral valvotomy is an option if required. Maternal mortality is reported at around 2 per cent and adverse fetal outcome is directly related to the severity of the stenosis.
See Chapter 12, *Obstetrics by Ten Teachers*, 19th edition.

38 F, T, T, F, T

It is important to test the partner for carrier status so that an accurate assessment of fetal risk can be made. The couple should be offered genetic counselling regarding the risk of the fetus having cystic fibrosis or being a carrier. Pancreatic function is affected in women with cystic fibrosis and 8 per cent will develop gestational diabetes in pregnancy. Ideally, vaginal delivery should be the aim; however, the second stage may be shortened in the event of maternal exhaustion. The fetal risks include fetal growth restriction.
See Chapter 12, *Obstetrics by Ten Teachers*, 19th edition.

39 T, F, T, T, T

Iron demand in pregnancy increases from 2 mg to 4 mg daily. The diagnosis of iron deficiency is suspected if the mean corpuscular volume (MCV) is below 85 fL. Low levels of serum iron and ferritin help to confirm the diagnosis. Nutritional status affects the iron stores, and repeated pregnancy and poor social factors may lead to anaemia, as will the increased iron requirements of multiple pregnancy. Blood transfusion should be avoided, if possible, because of the small risk of antibody production and transfusion reaction.

See Chapter 12, *Obstetrics by Ten Teachers*, 19th edition.

40 T, F, F, T, F

Carbamazepine is classically associated with neural tube defects. However, sodium valproate is associated with NTDs, genitourinary and cardiac defects, and phenytoin is associated with cardiac and genitourinary defects. Vitamin K supplementation should be recommended from 36 weeks' gestation. This is because vitamin K-dependent clotting factors within the newborn may be reduced and lead to haemorrhagic disease. Although magnesium sulphate is the treatment of choice for an undiagnosed seizure during labour, intravenous benzodiazepines (i.e. lorazepam, carbamazepine) are the recognized treatment for status epilepticus during labour.

See Chapter 12, *Obstetrics by Ten Teachers*, 19th edition.

41 T, T, T, T, T

Congenital cytomegalovirus (CMV) is associated with various fetal manifestations. These include hepatosplenomegaly, microcephaly, intrauterine growth retardation, hyperbilirubinaemia, intracerebral calcification and mental retardation. Only 5–10 per cent of infants will be symptomatic at birth. Congenital CMV is a cause of fetal hydrops and, as such, polyhydramnios.

See Chapter 13, *Obstetrics by Ten Teachers*, 19th edition.

42 F, T, T, F, T

Toxoplasmosis during the first trimester of pregnancy is most likely to cause fetal damage, but transmission to the fetus occurs in only 10–25 per cent of cases. In the third trimester, 75–90 per cent of infections are transmitted, but the risk of fetal damage is almost zero at term. Fetal varicella syndrome occurs in a minority of infected fetuses (approximately 1 per cent). No case of fetal varicella syndrome has been reported when maternal infection has occurred after 28 weeks. Up to 70 per cent of fetuses become infected if the mother has primary or secondary syphilis during pregnancy; however, the spectrum of congenital disease varies greatly.

See Chapter 13, *Obstetrics by Ten Teachers*, 19th edition.

43 T, T, F, T, T

Human immunodeficiency virus (HIV) is a retrovirus, with the genetic code in a single strand of RNA. Vertical transmission occurs in 25–30 per cent of pregnancies where there is no intervention to reduce the risk. Three interventions have been shown to reduce the vertical transmission of HIV. These are: (1) avoiding breastfeeding; (2) elective Caesarean section; and (3) antiviral medication during the latter half of pregnancy. If all three interventions are undertaken, then the risk of transmission is probably less than 3 per cent. Elective vaginal delivery can be considered if the mother is taking triple drug antiretroviral therapy and has a viral load of less than 50 copies/mL at the time of delivery. In this case, obstetric interventions such as scalp electrodes and fetal blood sampling should be avoided.

See Chapter 13, *Obstetrics by Ten Teachers*, 19th edition.

44 F, T, F, T, T

The pudendal nerve passes behind and below the ischial spine. The pelvic inlet is defined as the area bounded in front by the symphysis pubis, on each side by the upper margin of the pubic bone, the ileopectineal line and the ala of the sacrum, and posteriorly by the promontory of the sacrum. The normal anterior–posterior diameter of the pelvic inlet is 11 cm and the transverse diameter is 13.5 cm. The AP diameter of the pelvic outlet is 13.5 cm, with a transverse diameter of 11 cm. The normal angle of the inlet is 60° to the horizontal; however, in Afro-Caribbean women, this angle may be as much as 90°.

See Chapter 14, *Obstetrics by Ten Teachers*, 19th edition.

45 T, F, F, T, T

The anterior fontanelle is diamond shaped and is formed at the junction of the sagittal, frontal and coronal sutures. The sutures of the vault are soft unossified membranes, whereas the sutures of the face and the skull base are firmly united. The longitudinal diameter of the vertex presentation is the suboccipital–bregmatic diameter. The occipito-mental diameter is 13 cm and describes the brow presentation. This is usually too large to pass through the maternal pelvis.

See Chapter 14, *Obstetrics by Ten Teachers*, 19th edition.

46 F, F, T, T, F

Progress in labour is measured by dilation of the cervix and descent of the presenting part. Progress may be satisfactory in the absence of strong frequent contractions or may be unsatisfactory even when contractions are strong. Rupture of the membranes can occur before the onset of labour or may not occur until shortly before delivery.

See Chapter 14, *Obstetrics by Ten Teachers*, 19th edition.

47 F, F, T, T, T

Engagement is said to have occurred when the widest part of the presenting part has passed through the pelvic inlet. Restitution occurs directly after delivery of the fetal head, allowing the fetal head to align itself with the shoulders in the oblique position. In order to deliver, the shoulders then have to rotate from the oblique into the AP plane. During this rotation, the fetal occiput rotates to the transverse and this is termed external rotation.

See Chapter 14, *Obstetrics by Ten Teachers*, 19th edition.

48 F, T, F, T, F

Face presentation occurs in about 1 in 500 labours. Rarely, extension of the neck can be due to a fetal anomaly, such as a thyroid tumour. If progress in labour is excellent, and the chin remains mento-anterior, vaginal delivery is possible by flexion. Oxytocin should not be used and, if there are any concerns about fetal condition, Caesarean section should be carried out.

See Chapter 14, *Obstetrics by Ten Teachers*, 19th edition.

49 T, T, F, F, T

The Bishop score relates to the favourability of the cervix for induction of labour. It scores the station of the presenting part, the cervical consistency, position, dilatation and effacement. High scores are associated with an easier, shorter induction that is less likely to fail. Low scores are associated with longer inductions of labour, which are more likely to fail and result in Caesarean section.

See Chapter 14, *Obstetrics by Ten Teachers*, 19th edition.

50 F, F, T, T, T

Brow presentation is the least common malpresentation (1 in 2000), not the least common malposition. The eyes, nose and mouth will be palpable in a face presentation. In a brow presentation, the anterior fontanelle, supraorbital ridges and nose will be palpable. The presenting diameter is the wide (13 cm) mento-vertical diameter. Brow presentation is incompatible with vaginal delivery and Caesarean section will be required.

See Chapter 14, *Obstetrics by Ten Teachers*, 19th edition.

51 T, F, T, F, T

Any cause of antepartum haemorrhage may also present with bleeding in the first stage of labour, including a placenta praevia or intrapartum abruption. To these must be added conditions occurring in the first stage of labour. Vaginal trauma usually occurs in the second stage with delivery of the fetal head.

See Chapter 14, *Obstetrics by Ten Teachers*, 19th edition.

52 F, T, T, F, T

Kielland's forceps have a cephalic curve and lack a pelvic curve to allow rotation within the genital tract. The sliding lock is used to correct asynclitism. Kielland's forceps should not be applied to a high head (one that is more than one-fifth palpable abdominally). The minimum analgesia requirement for delivery by Kielland's forceps is an effective epidural or a spinal block. Kielland's forceps should be used only by an experienced operator.

See Chapter 15, *Obstetrics by Ten Teachers*, 19th edition.

53 T, T, T, T, T

Difficulty with delivery of the fetal shoulder is termed shoulder dystocia. The incidence varies between 0.2 per cent and 1.2 per cent depending on the definition used. Risk factors for shoulder dystocia include large baby, small mother, maternal obesity, post-maturity and assisted vaginal delivery. Shoulder dystocia should be managed in a sequence of manoeuvres designed to facilitate delivery without fetal damage. The first of these manoeuvres is McRobert's manoeuvre (maximal flex and abduction of the patient's hips onto her abdomen) and this will effect safe delivery in approximately 90 per cent of cases. Fundal pressure should be avoided, as it may lead to rupture of the uterus. Inappropriate traction on the fetal head causing lateral flexion should be avoided, as this can result in nerve damage and Erb's palsy.

See Chapter 16, *Obstetrics by Ten Teachers*, 19th edition.

54 T, F, T, F, T

Pre-eclampsia can manifest in a multitude of ways, presenting with symptoms ranging from vaginal bleeding (from placental abruption) to a tonic-clonic seizure. There are, however, some characteristic symptoms that should be screened for in all patients in whom the diagnosis is suspected. Flashing lights in the vision, epigastric pain and restlessness are all symptoms that warrant prompt investigation. Sleepiness and rash are not characteristic of the disorder.

See Chapter 16, *Obstetrics by Ten Teachers*, 19th edition.

55 T, F, F, T, F

Severe postpartum haemorrhage is a life-threatening condition, to which a prompt co-ordinated response is essential. Senior obstetric, anaesthetic and midwifery personnel should be requested to attend urgently. Haematology input should be requested, but it is rare that they will need to attend labour ward, and will be more effective co-ordinating the blood bank response. Facial oxygen is a standard part of basic resuscitative measures. IV fluid will help replace blood loss and maintain blood pressure, but wide-bore peripheral IV access will be more easily gained and equally effective. Ultrasound scan of the uterus may be useful in identifying problems such as retained products of conception, but will not form part of the initial management.

See Chapter 16, *Obstetrics by Ten Teachers*, 19th edition.

56 T, T, T, F, F

Resuscitation of the pregnant woman requires some additional steps for maximal efficacy. The abdomen should be tilted (for example with a Cardiff wedge) to relieve caval compression and increase venous return. The weight of the mammary glands increases in late gestation and may alter the pressures required to achieve adequate ventilation. The functional lung capacity is reduced, however, and the diaphragm may be splinted by the gravid uterus. The lower oesophageal sphincter is relaxed due to hormonal effects in pregnancy and

therefore aspiration is more likely if the airway is not protected. If initial resuscitative efforts are not successful by 4 minutes after cardiac output is lost, then a perimortem Caesarean section should be performed, primarily to increase the chances of successful maternal resuscitation.
See Chapter 16, *Obstetrics by Ten Teachers*, 19th edition.

57 F, T, T, F, F

The major constituents of breast milk are lactose, protein, fat and water. Relative to cow's milk, human milk contains more lactose and less protein. Breast milk contains less iron than formula or cow's milk, but it is more readily absorbed from the gut. All vitamins other than vitamin K are found in breast milk; routine supplementation is therefore given to neonates at birth. Breastfeeding is associated with a reduction in atopic illness.
See Chapter 17, *Obstetrics by Ten Teachers*, 19th edition.

58 T, F, T, T, F

Prolonged rupture of the membranes increases the risk of ascending infection via the genital tract, as does a prolonged second stage. Operative delivery (whether vaginal or abdominal) carries a higher risk than spontaneous delivery. If the membranes are not ruptured then there is no increased risk associated with prolonged pregnancy. Home birth is not associated with a higher infection risk than hospital delivery.
See Chapter 17, *Obstetrics by Ten Teachers*, 19th edition.

59 T, T, F, T, T

Average blood loss is higher after instrumental delivery than spontaneous delivery. Perineal pain may be due to increased spontaneous tears, haematoma formation or episiotomy repair. Mastitis is not more common following an instrumental delivery. Obstetric palsy may be due to exaggerated lithotomy position during instrumental delivery. Puerperal infection is more common where instrumentation of the genital tract has occurred.
See Chapter 17, *Obstetrics by Ten Teachers*, 19th edition.

60 T, T, F, F, F

Post-natal blues may represent a response to the fluctuations in hormone levels post-delivery. In prolonged or severe cases post-natal depression must be considered. Treatment of anaemia may help to shorten the course. The phenomenon is more often seen in women who have had Caesarean sections.
See Chapter 18, *Obstetrics by Ten Teachers*, 19th edition.

61 T, F, T, F, F

Mental illness can relapse or be exacerbated in pregnancy, therefore it is important to screen for a personal or family history of mental illness. There is a theoretical risk of teratogenicity from psychotropic medication, but this may be outweighed by the chance of relapse. Inpatient care post-natally should be facilitated in a mother and baby unit if possible.
See Chapter 18, *Obstetrics by Ten Teachers*, 19th edition.

62 T, T, T, F, T

Two-thirds of babies develop jaundice in the week 1 of life. Any visible jaundice in the first 24 hours must be urgently investigated and assumed to represent haemolysis unless proven otherwise. Ebstein's anomaly is a cardiac malformation and not associated with neonatal jaundice.
See Chapter 19, *Obstetrics by Ten Teachers*, 19th edition.

63 F, T, T, F, F

Vitamin K is offered at birth to all babies in the UK. Late-onset vitamin K deficiency bleeding (VKDB) can be prevented with a single intramuscular dose of vitamin K. While repeated oral doses may be an alternative to intramuscular dosing, a single oral dose is less effective in preventing late-onset VKDB. Early-onset

VKDB is seen in babies whose mothers were on medication that interferes with the production of vitamin K-dependent clotting factors. Classical VKDB presents on days 2–7 with bleeding from the umbilical stump, bruising or melaena.

See Chapter 19, *Obstetrics by Ten Teachers*, 19th edition.

64 F, T, T, F, T

Neonatal resuscitation requires around 90 compressions and 30 breaths per minute (3:1 ratio). The initial inflation breaths are given at higher pressure and for longer than subsequent maintenance breaths. Naloxone or blood transfusion may be considered by the attending paediatrician where appropriate.

See Chapter 19, *Obstetrics by Ten Teachers*, 19th edition.

65 T, F, T, T, F

Informed consent requires that the patient should be able to understand, retain and weigh the information given, and that they should be able to communicate their decision. There is no time limit imposed on informed consent, and quick decisions may be required in difficult situations on the labour ward. Verbal consent is adequate to carry out a procedure if time pressures demand this, but written documentation of consent is preferred where possible.

See Chapter 20, *Obstetrics by Ten Teachers*, 19th edition.

SINGLE BEST ANSWER QUESTIONS

QUESTIONS

Obstetric history taking and examination

1 **Which statement is correct regarding calculating expected date of delivery (EDD)?**
a) Pregnancy is dated from conception.
b) The last menstrual period (LMP) is reliable if the cycles are irregular.
c) The average length of pregnancy is 280 days.
d) LMP defined dates are more accurate than those calculated from USS.
e) Head circumference may be used to date a pregnancy until 25 weeks.

2 **Which best describes the reproductive history of a woman at 12/40 with a previous twin delivery and a stillbirth at 27/40?**
a) G3P3.
b) G3P4.
c) G4P4.
d) G4P3.
e) G4P2.

3 **Which statement is correct regarding general examination in pregnancy?**
a) The abdomen should always be palpated lying flat.
b) Breast examination should be conducted as part of routine antenatal care.
c) Approximately 80 per cent of women have an audible murmur at 12/40.
d) A symphysis–fundal height measurement should be plotted at every visit after 16/40.
e) Nipple examination can predict women who will need help in breastfeeding.

Normal fetal development and growth

4 **A woman is found to have oligohydramnios at 30/40. Which of the following is the most likely cause?**
a) Duodenal atresia.

b) Placental choriangioma.
c) Diabetes.
d) Oesophageal atresia.
e) Renal agenesis.

5   An infant is delivered at 27/40 and taken to the neonatal unit. Which problem is most likely to be experienced?
a) Incomplete formation of the epidermis from the mesoderm.
b) Excessive vernix formation.
c) Lanugo shedding.
d) Thermoregulation due to thin skin.
e) Lack of hair follicle development.

Antenatal care

6   A woman contacts her midwife with concerns regarding fetal well-being at 32/40 in a previously normal pregnancy. Which is the best management?
a) Auscultation of the fetal heart at home by midwife.
b) Encourage the patient to record a 24-hour kick chart.
c) Book a growth scan within 2 days.
d) Attend hospital if fetal movements are decreased.
e) Advise repeat nuchal translucency scan.

Antenatal imaging and assessment of fetal well-being

7   A thirty-seven-year-old woman attends for a routine dating scan. She asks you in detail what information will be obtained from the scan. Which of the following will not be possible?
a) Accurate dating of the pregnancy.
b) The detection of placenta praevia.
c) The early detection of twin pregnancies.
d) The detection of a failed pregnancy.
e) The detection of uterine abnormalities.

Prenatal diagnosis

8   Which option is correct regarding diagnostic ultrasound?
a) It employs the use of low-intensity, high-frequency sound waves.
b) Between 12 and 20 weeks, the crown rump length and the femur length are the most reproducible assessment of gestational age.
c) It can be used to determine chorionicity accurately in twin pregnancy at the 20/40 scan.
d) An increase in nuchal translucency is associated with cardiac defects.
e) In 6 per cent of pregnancies there will be a serious structural abnormality.

9   The obstetric doctor on call is asked to review a cardiotocograph performed prior to induction of labour in a 39/40 multigravida. Which of the following features should help to reassure the doctor that this is a normal trace?
a) The baseline heart rate is 100 beats per minute.
b) The baseline variability is <5 beats per minute.
c) An acceleration of 15 beats per minute for 15 seconds is present on the trace.

d) There are no significant accelerations of the fetal heart on the 30-minute recording.

e) The tocograph is picking up regular contractions.

10 Choose the best statement in regard to genetic counselling:

a) If no genetic basis is known for a condition, there is little use in genetic counselling for the parents.

b) Less anxiety is caused by performing a test as soon as possible and discussing the condition suspected with results available.

c) A discussion regarding termination should not be raised with the parents unless a test result has shown a serious condition.

d) A 1 per cent risk of miscarriage from an invasive test will be considered acceptable to all parents.

e) A consent form should be signed prior to genetic tests being carried out.

Antenatal obstetric complications

11 A twenty-fou-year-old IV drug user who smokes attends the antenatal clinic. She has continued to use heroin throughout her pregnancy, but has reduced her smoking. Which complication is she most likely to experience?

a) Placental abruption.

b) Cervical incompetence.

c) Neonatal withdrawal syndrome.

d) Antepartum haemorrhage.

e) Severe intrauterine growth restriction.

12 On routine antenatal bloods, a thirty-year-old woman is found to be Rhesus negative. Which piece of advice regarding the management of her pregnancy is correct?

a) Her fetus will also be Rhesus negative.

b) If there is concern later in pregnancy regarding vaginal bleeding then a Kleihauer test should be performed.

c) She should have a routine dose of anti-D at 23/40.

d) Once she has had two doses of anti-D, further administration will not be required.

e) If this pregnancy is not affected by Rhesus disease, there should be no problem in subsequent pregnancies.

Twins and higher multiple pregnancies

13 Which of the following is not an increased risk in multiple pregnancy?

a) Placenta praevia.

b) Diabetes mellitus.

c) Pre-eclampsia.

d) Malpresentation.

e) Intrauterine growth restriction (IUGR).

Late miscarriage and early birth

14 Which statement is most accurate regarding cervical cerclage?

a) In a high-risk patient it should be performed as soon as practical after confirmation of intrauterine pregnancy.

b) Is a suitable procedure in any woman with a history of delivery between 20 and 26 weeks.

c) Should be performed using an absorbable suture material.

d) May be placed using a transvaginal approach.

e) Requires a second anaesthetic procedure for removal when delivery is imminent.

Medical diseases complicating pregnancy

15 **You review a thirty-three-year-old woman with a history of congenital heart disease in the antenatal clinic. In making a plan for the management of her pregnancy, which step is least appropriate?**
a) Booking a detailed fetal cardiology scan.
b) Avoiding anaemia and prescribing supplementary iron if necessary.
c) Prophylactic antibiotics should operative delivery be required.
d) A birth pool to provide helpful extra analgesia.
e) May benefit from a shortened second stage of labour.

16 **Which of the following is correct regarding hyperthyroidism in pregnancy?**
a) Should be treated surgically rather than with carbimazole.
b) Can be diagnosed by total T4 measurements.
c) More than half are due to Grave's disease.
d) The main complications for the fetus include growth restriction and fetal bradycardia.
e) Therapy should maintain free T4 and T3 levels in the low normal range.

17 **A pregnant woman with gestational diabetes asks you about the increased risks to her fetus. You describe all of the following except:**
a) Polycythaemia.
b) Hypermagnesaemia.
c) Traumatic delivery.
d) Neonatal jaundice.
e) Hypoglycaemia.

18 **Which of the following is least accurate regarding adrenal disease in pregnancy?**
a) Cushing's syndrome may resemble the features of normal pregnancy.
b) Addison's disease may be difficult to diagnose in pregnancy due to changes in steroid profiles.
c) Phaeochromocytoma may be diagnosed using 24-hour urine catecholamine testing.
d) Steroid replacement therapy should be reduced to allow normal delivery.
e) Phaeochromocytoma may mimic the features of pre-eclampsia.

19 **The following are correct regarding thalassaemias except:**
a) They represent the most common genetic blood disorders.
b) They result from an amino acid substitution.
c) Alpha-thalassaemia major is incompatible with intrauterine life.
d) It is important to screen the partner.
e) Beta-thalassaemia minor is not a problem antenatally.

Perinatal infections

20 **You are counselling a pregnant woman in the antenatal clinic who has known hepatitis with regard to fetal risk. Which form of hepatitis has the highest rate of fetal transmission?**
a) Hepatitis A.
b) Hepatitis B.
c) Hepatitis C.
d) Hepatitis B+D.
e) Hepatitis E.

21 Choose the best option with regard to a non-immune pregnant woman with an exposure to chickenpox:
a) Should be given the varicella zoster vaccine as soon as possible after exposure.
b) Should be given varicella zoster immunoglobulin as soon as possible after exposure.
c) Does not need intervention unless symptoms of chickenpox occur.
d) Should not be treated with acyclovir in the third trimester.
e) Has a 15 per cent risk of having a baby with fetal varicella syndrome.

Labour

22 Choose the option that is the greatest contraindication to epidural anaesthesia:
a) Previous treatment with anticoagulants.
b) Multiple pregnancy.
c) Patients receiving narcotics.
d) Hypertension in pregnancy.
e) Hypovolaemia.

Operative intervention in obstetrics

23 Which of the following is the main advantage to performing a medio-lateral episiotomy?
a) Less blood loss.
b) Reduced incidence of dyspareunia.
c) Less anal sphincter damage.
d) Less pain in the postpartum period.
e) It is easier to repair.

24 As the obstetric SHO on call, you are preparing to perform a ventouse delivery. Which of the following is not mandatory to ensure?
a) Gestation less than 35 weeks.
b) The cervix is fully dilated.
c) Adequate maternal analgesia.
d) Empty bladder.
e) Fetal membranes are ruptured.

Obstetric emergencies

25 Choose the option that is less common after Caesarean delivery than after vaginal delivery:
a) Pulmonary embolism.
b) Postpartum haemorrhage.
c) Post-natal depression.
d) Amniotic fluid embolism.
e) Infection.

26 Which of the following reasons for performing Caesarean section contributes least to the total Caesarean section rate?
a) Malpresentation.
b) Placenta praevia.
c) Previous Caesarean section.
d) Dystocia.
e) Suspected fetal compromise.

27 Which of the following is not a factor classically implicated in postpartum haemorrhage?
a) Tone.
b) Trauma.
c) Tamponade.
d) Thrombin.
e) Tissue.

Psychiatric disorders and the puerperium

28 Which statement is true regarding mental illness in pregnancy?
a) The majority of women with postpartum psychiatric disorders have pre-existing mental illness.
b) In women with pre-existing psychiatric disorders, these usually improve during pregnancy.
c) The incidence of admission with puerperal psychosis is approximately 2 per cent.
d) Panic attacks should not be considered a feature of normal pregnancy.
e) Psychotropic drug therapies should be discontinued during pregnancy.

Neonatology

29 The components of the Apgar score include all except:
a) Appearance.
b) Pulse rate.
c) Good eye opening.
d) Activity.
e) Respiratory effort.

Ethical and medicolegal issues in obstetric practice

30 Which statement is not true regarding the regulations of the Abortion Act and Section 37 of the Human Fertilisation and Embryology Act?
a) The regulations dealing with emergency termination are in Sections F and G.
b) A termination at 26 weeks may be allowed in some circumstances under Section E.
c) Approximately 1 per cent of terminations in the UK are carried out under Section E.
d) The terms of the Abortion Act allow the interests of the pregnant woman's existing children to be taken into account.
e) The terms of the Abortion Act allow the interests of the pregnant woman's partner to be taken into account.

SBA ANSWERS

1 C

Pregnancy is historically dated from the last menstrual period. However, this assumes a 28-day cycle and may need to be adjusted if longer. Ultrasound dates are more accurate than the LMP. Head circumference is most appropriate for dating between 14 and 20 weeks.

See Chapter 1, *Obstetrics by Ten Teachers*, 19th edition.

2 A

Gravidity includes all pregnancies that the woman has had and any current pregnancy. Parity refers to all completed pregnancies that have progressed beyond 24 weeks, regardless of whether live or stillborn. Hence a twin pregnancy will represent G1 P2 if both babies are delivered after 24/40. The patient in question is in her third pregnancy (G3) and has delivered three babies at >24/40 (P3).

See Chapter 1, *Obstetrics by Ten Teachers*, 19th edition.

3 C

Many heavily pregnant women are uncomfortable lying flat and are best examined semirecumbent. Breast and nipple examination are unnecessary as part of routine antenatal care. Increased cardiac output causes flow murmurs in the majority of women by the end of the first trimester. Symphysis–fundal height is usually plotted beyond 24/40.

See Chapter 1, *Obstetrics by Ten Teachers*, 19th edition.

4 E

Amniotic fluid is initially secreted by the amnion, but is a transudate of fetal serum by week 10. After 16 weeks the skin becomes impermeable. Thereafter the increase in amniotic fluid relies on the fetal kidneys and lungs to produce fluid. A fetus renal agenesis will therefore suffer from oligo-or anhydramnios. Fetal swallowing helps to remove fluid and thus oesophageal and duodenal atresia are associated with polyhydramnios. Diabetes and placental chorioangioma are other causes of polyhydramnios.

See Chapter 4, *Obstetrics by Ten Teachers*, 19th edition.

5 D

The skin consists of two layers, the epidermis (derived from the ectoderm) and the dermis (derived from the mesoderm). The periderm produces a creamy protective layer known as the vernix, which rubs off after birth. Lanugo is usually shed before birth. Hair follicles normally develop between 12 and 16/40, hence this should not be a problem for this infant. Thermoregulation, dehydration and infection, however, are all important issues associated with the skin of premature infants.

See Chapter 4, *Obstetrics by Ten Teachers*, 19th edition.

6 D

Routine auscultation of the fetal heart is often performed at midwifery appointments for reassurance, but if there is genuine cause for concern, such as reduced fetal movements, then the woman should be evaluated in a hospital setting. Women do not need to keep records of fetal movements, but should seek further care if the movements are significantly reduced. Growth scans are not performed in normal antenatal care unless there is a specific concern or indication. The nuchal translucency test is offered to all women at 11–14 weeks and there are no data to validate use outside this period.

See Chapter 5, *Obstetrics by Ten Teachers*, 19th edition.

7 B

Early ultrasound is more accurate in dating the pregnancy than use of LMP. Placental site is first evaluated at 20/40, with follow-up scans if it is low-lying. Twin pregnancy is detected at the dating scan and may be the best opportunity to determine the chorionicity of the pregnancy. Uterine abnormalities such as bicornuate uterus are often best seen at this stage before the cavity becomes too distended.

See Chapter 6, *Obstetrics by Ten Teachers*, 19th edition.

8 D

The technique of ultrasound uses high-frequency, low-intensity sound waves to generate an image. Fetal age can be assessed accurately prior to 12 weeks by measuring the crown–rump length and from 12 to 20 weeks' gestation can be determined from biparietal diameter. The chorionicity of twin pregnancy is best determined in the first trimester; this should ideally occur at approximately 12 weeks. Nuchal translucency has been shown to be a screening test for Down's syndrome, other chromosomal abnormalities and cardiac defects. Serious fetal structural abnormalities are diagnosed in 3 per cent of all pregnancies.

See Chapter 6, *Obstetrics by Ten Teachers*, 19th edition.

9 C

The normal fetal heart rate at term is 110–150 bpm, while prior to term 160 bpm is the upper limit of normal. Normal baseline variability reflects a normal fetal autonomic system. Baseline variability is considered reduced when it is <5 bpm. The presence of two or more accelerations on a 20–30-minute cardiotocogram defines a reactive trace. The tocograph gives no indication of fetal well-being.

See Chapter 6, *Obstetrics by Ten Teachers*, 19th edition.

10 E

Even if the aetiology of a condition is not fully understood, the parents of an affected child will still benefit from follow-up and discussion prior to subsequent pregnancies. No test should be performed without a full discussion of the information that the results will yield and all the options that may then be available. Informed consent is a vital part of the process of genetic testing and it is good practice to record this as a formal record. Many parents will consider a 1 per cent risk of miscarriage acceptable to yield diagnostic information about the pregnancy, but it will not be acceptable to all couples. Prior to testing or diagnosis, the parents should be aware of the options available to them.

See Chapter 7, *Obstetrics by Ten Teachers*, 19th edition.

11 C

Fetal growth restriction is a consequence of tobacco, alcohol and cocaine use during pregnancy. Growth restriction relates to smoking in a dose-dependent manner, hence severe growth restriction is unlikely if smoking has been drastically reduced. Opioids and cocaine use carry a risk of preterm labour. Placental abruption is associated with alcohol and cocaine use. Reducing the dose of opioids suddenly during pregnancy can precipitate withdrawal in both the mother and the fetus, and the fetus is susceptible after birth if the possibility is not recognized and prepared for.

See Chapter 8, *Obstetrics by Ten Teachers*, 19th edition.

12 B

Approximately 15 per cent of the Caucasian population are Rhesus negative. The Rhesus status of the fetus depends also on the partner's blood type. Exogenous anti-D immunoglobulin is administered in an attempt to prevent the manufacture of endogenous antibody by the mother, as this would sensitize the immune system and put subsequent fetuses at risk. Routine doses of anti-D are usually given at 28 and 34 weeks, but it should be considered after every sensitizing event. The Kleihauer test determines the proportion of fetal cells within the maternal circulation and hence helps determine anti-D dosage.

See Chapter 8, *Obstetrics by Ten Teachers*, 19th edition.

13 A

All the physiological changes of pregnancy are exacerbated in multiple pregnancy. The greater placental area makes placenta praevia and pre-eclampsia more likely. It has been a subject of debate whether gestational diabetes is more common in multiple pregnancies, but recent studies have failed to find any evidence that the risk is increased.

See Chapter 9, *Obstetrics by Ten Teachers*, 19th edition.

14 D

Cervical cerclage should be considered in a small group of carefully selected patients. Studies suggest benefit in women with a history of three or more late miscarriages of preterm deliveries. It is best performed after 12–14 weeks to avoid the problems of early pregnancy loss and to assess nuchal translucency prior to intervention. The most common suture material is a Mercilene tape. Transvaginal or transabdominal approaches are possible. A McDonald suture can usually be removed without recourse to regional anaesthesia.

See Chapter 11, *Obstetrics by Ten Teachers*, 19th edition.

15 D

The incidence of congenital heart disease in the general population is 8 per 1000 live births. However, if the parent is affected, the incidence raises to 5 per 100 live births; therefore, all pregnant women with congenital heart disease should have a detailed fetal cardiology scan. The haemodynamic changes of pregnancy increase the strain on the heart. Anaemia exacerbates this situation. Dysrhythmias occur in less than 3 per cent of women. However, they require urgent treatment. Prophylactic antibiotics should be given to any women with congenital heart defects.

See Chapter 12, *Obstetrics by Ten Teachers*, 19th edition.

16 C

Hyperthyroidism in pregnancy is treated pharmacologically. Radioactive iodine is contraindicated due to the effect on the fetal thyroid gland. The diagnosis of hyperthyroidism in pregnancy requires increased free T3 and T4, with reduced levels of thyroid-stimulating hormone (TSH). Approximately 90 per cent of cases of hyperthyroidism in pregnancy are due to Grave's disease. Levels of free T3/T4 in pregnancy should be maintained in the high normal range. The main risks to the fetus are of growth restriction, stillbirth, fetal tachycardia and premature delivery.

See Chapter 12, *Obstetrics by Ten Teachers*, 19th edition.

17 B

The infant of a diabetic mother is exposed to various metabolic insults. There is an increased risk of hypoglycaemia, hypocalcaemia and hypomagnesaemia after birth. Macrosomia carries an increased risk of traumatic delivery.

See Chapter 12, *Obstetrics by Ten Teachers*, 19th edition.

18 D

Increased levels of steroid hormones are normal in pregnancy, and the effects of these may be similar to those of Cushing's syndrome – striae, weight gain and glucose intolerance in particular. A 24-hour urine catecholamine measurement combined with imaging of the adrenal glands provides the diagnosis of phaeochromocytoma. The sudden increases in blood pressure with headache, blurred vision and anxiety that are typical of phaeochromocytoma may be mistaken for the more common syndrome of pre-eclampsia. During normal labour steroid replacement therapy is increased to account for the additional physiological stress.

See Chapter 12, *Obstetrics by Ten Teachers*, 19th edition.

19 B

The thalassaemia syndromes are the most common genetic blood disorders. Sickle cell disease is caused by a single amino acid substitution, but thalassaemias lead to a reduced production of normal haemoglobin. If the partner is also affected then the chances of the fetus having alpha-thalassaemia is 1 in 4. Alpha-thalassaemia major is lethal.

See Chapter 12, *Obstetrics by Ten Teachers*, 19th edition.

20 B

Hepatitis A and E represent acute infectious disease. The incidence of hepatitis A in pregnancy is 1 in 1000 and fetal transmission is extremely rare. Hepatitis E has a higher chance of causing fulminant hepatitic failure in pregnancy, but no cases of fetal transmission have been reported. The prevalence of hepatitis C in pregnant women is estimated at 1–2 per cent and the rate of fetal transmission at 5–10 per cent. There is no evidence that hepatitis B is more common in pregnancy; 20–30 per cent of fetuses will be affected. There are a few cases reported of co-transmission of hepatitis B and D.

See Chapter 12, *Obstetrics by Ten Teachers*, 19th edition.

21 B

Pregnant women should have varicella zoster virus IgG measured if they are exposed to chickenpox during pregnancy. Non-immune women with a significant exposure should receive VZV immunoglobulin as soon as possible. Oral aciclovir is an appropriate treatment for women with symptoms who are beyond 20/40. The clinical course of chickenpox tends to be more severe in the pregnant population. Fetal varicella syndrome occurs in approximately 1 per cent of affected fetuses.

See Chapter 13, *Obstetrics by Ten Teachers*, 19th edition.

22 E

Epidural anaesthesia is an effective means of pain relief in labour. Certain conditions make epidural anaesthesia advantageous, including maternal hypertension (as it tends to decrease blood pressure). Conversely, where the blood pressure is already low (for example hypovolaemia), epidural anaesthesia is contraindicated. In labours where there is a high chance of operative intervention, for example multiple gestations, epidural anaesthesia may be advantageous.

See Chapter 14, *Obstetrics by Ten Teachers*, 19th edition.

23 C

In the UK, where episiotomy is required it is usually cut medio-lateral. This reduces the incidence of extension of the cut to involve the anal sphincter. This risk of involving the sphincter is higher if a midline episiotomy is cut; however, cutting in the midline has the advantages of less bleeding, less pain and an easier repair.

See Chapter 15, *Obstetrics by Ten Teachers*, 19th edition.

24 A

Ventouse delivery is contraindicated in gestations below 35/40 and in face or breech presentations. Ventouse can be applied only when the cervix is fully dilated and the fetal membranes are ruptured. Where sufficient maternal effort is possible, it is an appropriate strategy in cases of delay or fetal distress in the second stage. The maternal bladder should always be empty before instrumental delivery is attempted and adequate analgesia is a pre-requisite.

See Chapter 15, *Obstetrics by Ten Teachers*, 19th edition.

25 D

Caesarean section carries risks common to all operations, such as venous thromboembolism and infection. In addition the incidence of postpartum haemorrhage and post-natal depression is increased. Amniotic fluid embolism is a rare catastrophe, but may be associated with prolonged active pushing, especially with unruptured membranes.

See Chapters 15 and 16, *Obstetrics by Ten Teachers*, 19th edition.

26 B

There are many indications for Caesarean section, and all the factors listed are potential reasons for performing a Caesarean section. However, four major risk factors account for more than 70 per cent of Caesarean sections: previous Caesarean section, dystocia, malpresentation, suspected acute fetal compromise.

See Chapter 15, *Obstetrics by Ten Teachers*, 19th edition.

27 C

In assessing a patient with postpartum haemorrhage, the obstetrician should consider the '4 Ts' most likely to be responsible: Tone (of the uterus post-delivery), Trauma (to the vagina and soft tissues), Thrombin (coagulopathies) and Tissue (for example retained placenta).

See Chapter 16, *Obstetrics by Ten Teachers*, 19th edition.

28 D

More than 80 per cent of women with postpartum psychiatric disease will be suffering from their first-ever psychiatric illness. Women with pre-existing psychiatric disorders often experience an exacerbation or recurrence. The incidence admission with puerperal psychosis is 0.2 per cent, although 2 per cent of women will require referral to a psychiatrist in the puerperium. In many women established on psychotropic medication, the real risk of disease relapse on stopping outweighs the theoretical risks of fetal exposure.

See Chapter 18, *Obstetrics by Ten Teachers*, 19th edition.

29 C

The Apgar score is a tool that assists in recognition of the infant who is failing to make a successful transition to extrauterine life. It has five components, each of which is assigned a value 0, 1 or 2. The five original components are appearance, pulse rate, grimace, activity and respiratory effort. Eye opening is not assessed.

See Chapter 19, *Obstetrics by Ten Teachers*, 19th edition.

30 E

Abortion is legal in the UK provided that two doctors certify that the case satisfies one of the five grounds set out in the regulations of the Abortion Act and Section 37 of the Human Fertilisation and Embryology Act. Section E deals with cases where the fetus is likely to suffer from such 'physical or mental abnormalities as to be seriously handicapped'. It does not specify any particular abnormalities or gestation. In the UK 1 per cent of terminations are carried out under this regulation. The terms of Section D allow consideration of the existing child(ren) of the family of the pregnant woman. The interests of the partner are not specified in the Abortion Act.

See Chapter 20, *Obstetrics by Ten Teachers*, 19th edition

SHORT ANSWER QUESTIONS

QUESTIONS

Obstetric history taking and examination

1 Describe the features of the obstetric history that will influence management of subsequent pregnancies.
Obstetric histories should begin by stating the age, gravidity/parity and current gestation of the patient. Number and outcome of previous pregnancies are often summarized using gravidity and parity (GX,PY), although it may be more useful to describe in detail what has happened, especially if the history is complex.   (1 mark)

Early pregnancy complications are important to record, as recurrent miscarriage increases the risk of fetal loss and growth restriction. The use of assisted conception techniques may influence the subsequent course of the pregnancy, as donor gametes increase the chance of developing pre-eclampsia, and women may require increased support during pregnancy. Legally, the history of assisted conception should not be recorded without written permission from the patient.   (2 marks)

Previous maternal complications of pregnancy including pre-eclampsia and gestational diabetes carry a risk of recurrence and will often prompt increased monitoring during subsequent pregnancies, including early glucose tolerance testing.   (1 mark)

Fetal problems including growth restriction, congenital abnormalities and preterm delivery should all be noted. Previous preterm delivery increases the chance of a second preterm delivery. Previous intrauterine growth restriction will often prompt measurement of umbilical artery Doppler flow in the third trimester and extra ultrasound scans. Congenital abnormalities will usually require referral to a genetic counsellor to discuss the recurrence risk in detail.   (3 marks)

Late pregnancy and intrapartum problems are important for managing future pregnancies. Placental abruption has an increased risk of recurrence. Previous delivery by Caesarean section may influence planning for subsequent deliveries. Previous Caesarean section carries an increased risk of placenta praevia, uterine rupture and intraoperative complications if a repeat Caesarean section is performed.   (3 marks)

See Chapter 1, *Obstetrics by Ten Teachers*, 19th edition.

Modern maternity care

2 Discuss how maternity care has changed since its inception.

The modern National Health Service (NHS) was established by an Act of Parliament in 1946. This bill instigated free maternity care for all women. (1 mark)

Antenatal care was perceived as beneficial, acceptable and available for all. This was reinforced by the finding that the perinatal mortality rate seemed to be inversely proportional to the number of antenatal visits. (2 marks)

The co-operation card was launched on the NHS maternity services in the 1950s. This allowed a continuous record to be held by the mother and improved the communication between all health-care professionals involved in the delivery of maternity care. (2 marks)

The advent of obstetric ultrasound brought with it a dramatic revolution in the antenatal care and screening for fetal anomalies. This has allowed early pregnancy viability and accurate dating of pregnancies. Improved technologies with ultrasound have given rise to fetal anomaly screening. (3 marks)

During the early 1950s, there was a move towards hospital confinement from home confinement. Home deliveries are now an infrequent event with a countrywide average of about 2 per cent. (2 marks)

As new technology became available to monitor and induce labour in the late 1960s and early 1970s, the rate of induction of labour increased. Consumer groups such as the National Childbirth Trust began to question the efficacy of many interventions. (2 marks)

New standards in maternity care continue to be set, with government reports such as Changing Childbirth (1993) and Maternity Matters (2009) laying out targets and standards for childbirth in the UK. (1 mark)

See Chapter 2, *Obstetrics by Ten Teachers*, 19th edition.

Physiological changes in pregnancy

3 Outline the physiological changes that occur in response to pregnancy in the cardiovascular system, the cervix and the respiratory system.

Cardiovascular system

Early pregnancy is characterized by a decrease in the peripheral vascular resistance. A significant increase in the heart rate is observed as early as 5 weeks, and this contributes to an increase in cardiac output. This increase in heart rate continues into the third trimester. The stroke volume increases in the late first trimester and further increases the cardiac output. Blood pressure falls in the second trimester, but is comparable to the non-pregnant state by full term. (4 marks)

Cervix

Under the influence of the pregnancy hormones oestradiol and progesterone, the cervix becomes swollen and softer during pregnancy. Oestradiol stimulates the growth of the columnar epithelium of the cervical canal and this becomes visualized as an ectropion. The mucus glands become distended. Increased vascularity of the cervix causes it to become a blueish colour. Prostaglandins induce remodelling of the cervical collagen towards term, which allows softening. (4 marks)

Respiratory system

Dramatic changes occur in the respiratory system with the onset of pregnancy. The increased cardiac output causes a substantial increase in the pulmonary blood flow. There is an increase in the tidal volume. These two effects combine to give more efficient oxygen exchange. This increase in oxygen exchange causes a decrease in pCO_2 and a slight increase in pO_2. Thus oxygen availability to the tissues increases. The mechanical changes that occur in the lung include increases in the tidal volume, and decreases in the vital capacity and functional residual capacity in late pregnancy, due to the volume of the gravid uterus.   (4 marks)

See Chapter 3, *Obstetrics by Ten Teachers*, 19th edition.

Normal fetal development and growth

4 Write short notes on the fetal cardiovascular system and fetal blood.

Fetal cardiovascular system
The fetal circulation is significantly different from that of the adult. The lungs do not participate in oxygen exchange; therefore, their blood supply is significantly reduced. This reduction is achieved via the ductus arteriosus, which shunts blood away from the pulmonary artery and into the aorta.   (3 marks)

All oxygenation occurs within the placenta; therefore, blood passing back from the placenta via the umbilical vein needs to pass directly into the left side of the circulation. This is achieved in two ways. First, the ductus venous is present within the liver to direct blood into the right atrium of the heart. Second, the foramen ovale shunts oxygenated blood from the right atrium into the left atrium. Blood returns to the placenta for gaseous exchange via the umbilical arteries.   (3 marks)

Fetal blood
The first fetal blood cells are formed on the surface of the yolk sac and haemopoiesis continues at this site until the third month. During the fifth week of life, extramedullary haemopoiesis begins in the liver and, finally, bone marrow production starts at 7–8 weeks and reaches its peak by the 26th week of life.   (3 marks)

Haemoglobin F (HbF) is the most common in the fetus. HbF contains two alpha chains and two gamma chains, as opposed to adult haemoglobin which has two alpha chains with either two beta (HbA) or two delta (HbA2). HbF has a higher affinity for oxygen than adult haemoglobin (HbA), therefore enhancing oxygen transfer in the direction of the fetus across the placenta. The production of HbA is initiated at around 28 weeks and by term it makes up 20 per cent of the blood haemoglobin.   (3 marks)

See Chapter 4, *Obstetrics by Ten Teachers*, 19th edition.

Antenatal care

5 Write short notes on booking blood investigations, antenatal visit examination and customized antenatal care.

Blood tests
All pregnant women should be encouraged to undergo screening for a number of health issues. The following blood tests are normally performed. A full blood count is taken to screen for anaemia and thrombocytopenia. The woman's blood group and red-cell antibodies are also determined. If the woman is Rhesus negative, then she will be offered prophylactic anti-D administration at 28 and 32 weeks' gestation. Screening for haemoglobinopathies is also performed. Maternal blood will be screened for hepatitis B, HIV, rubella and syphilis. If any of these are positive, then appropriate treatment is initiated. In the case of HIV, this includes commencing antiviral drugs, advising against breastfeeding and offering Caesarean section. If hepatitis B infection is detected, and the patient is a carrier or has had a recent infection, then the fetus should be actively and passively immunized at birth. Women who are non-immune to rubella should be strongly counselled to avoid contact with suspected infection during pregnancy, and to be vaccinated postpartum. Syphilis is treated with high-dose maternal antibiotics.   (5 marks)

Antenatal visit examination

At each visit, the mother's blood pressure is tested to screen for pre-eclampsia. The maternal abdomen is palpated to confirm fetal presentation from approximately 32/40. The symphysis–fundal height is measured to screen fetal growth at visits after 25/40 and plotted on a chart.   (3 marks)

Customized antenatal care

Through the process of booking and antenatal care it may become apparent that a woman and her pregnancy have risk factors that are not met by standard services. In these cases, referral to other caregivers may be appropriate to ensure that the woman has customized antenatal care. One example of this is diabetes, where women receive customized care within a dedicated clinic. Women with risk factors in pregnancy should have care from a named consultant. Multidisciplinary care may be required, including from physicians, specialist midwives and genetic counsellors.   (4 marks)

See Chapter 5, *Obstetrics by Ten Teachers*, 19th edition.

Antenatal imaging and assessment of fetal well-being

6 Describe the use of ultrasound in obstetrics.

Ultrasound scanning is one of the most commonly used modalities in obstetrics. It can be carried out throughout all gestations from the time of gestational sac formation to assess the fetus and surrounding structures.   (1 mark)

In the first trimester, it is used to confirm viability, for accurate dating, and the diagnosis of twin pregnancies. It is also used for the determination of chorionicity in twin pregnancies. Uterine abnormalities and ovarian cysts may be determined during the first trimester scan. Within the first trimester, there is opportunity for ultrasound screening with the nuchal translucency between 11 and 13+6/40.   (4 marks)

During the second trimester, the anomaly scan is performed. This is undertaken at approximately 18–22 weeks. It involves a detailed structural survey of the fetus to detect any abnormalities. Uterine artery Doppler scans may be performed to determine whether the mother has an increased risk of developing pre-eclampsia. Cervical length may also be determined and used to assess the risk of preterm labour. Monochorionic twins may be assessed for signs of twin–twin transfusion.   (5 marks)

During the third trimester, ultrasound can be used to determine the placental site accurately. However, the most important role of ultrasound during the third trimester is that of determining fetal well-being. This is achieved by the measurement of fetal growth parameters, liquor volume and umbilical artery Doppler measurements.   (4 marks)

See Chapter 6, *Obstetrics by Ten Teachers*, 19th edition.

Prenatal diagnosis

7 Describe the techniques used for invasive prenatal diagnosis.

Amniocentesis is the most commonly used diagnostic test and can be performed from 15 weeks to term. It is carried out in pregnancies that have been identified as high risk by prior screening or history.   (2 marks)

Amniocentesis is performed with a transabdominal needle and carries fetal loss rates of 0.5–1.5 per cent. Fetal cells can be cultured from the fluid obtained and a karyotype determined.   (2 marks)

Chorionic villus sampling is an alternative to amniocentesis. It is also performed because of the increased risk on screening. However, it has the advantage that it can be performed either transabdominally or transvaginally from 11 weeks' gestation to term.   (2 marks)

CVS has a similar fetal loss rate to that of amniocentesis. One of the major disadvantages of CVS is the potential for contamination of the sample by maternal cells or the presence of placental mosaicism; this can make the result difficult to interpret. (2 marks)

Cordocentesis is the final method of invasive fetal testing. This involves the direct sampling of fetal blood from the umbilical vein. It is performed when a sample of fetal blood is required, for example to determine platelet count in alloimmune thrombocytopaenia. The test is usually performed at or after 20 weeks' gestation. (2 marks)

See Chapter 7, *Obstetrics by Ten Teachers*, 19th edition.

Antenatal obstetric complications

8 A twenty six-year-old woman presents in clinic at 30 weeks' gestation. The community midwife has referred her because she is 'large for dates'. An ultrasound scan has demonstrated polyhydramnios. Discuss the possible causes of polyhydramnios in this pregnancy.
The causes of polyhydramnios can be divided into maternal, fetal and placental. The aim of any investigation of polyhydramnios is to establish a diagnosis, so that a prognosis can be determined. (2 marks)

Initially a full maternal history should be taken. This should include medical history, as there are various diseases that can cause fetal polyhydramnios. The most common maternal disease associated with polyhydramnios is poorly controlled diabetes mellitus. Therefore, a random blood glucose level should be obtained and this should be followed by an oral glucose tolerance test, if indicated. Maternal red-cell antibodies should be checked to exclude isoimmunization, as this is associated with fetal hydrops. (4 marks)

A detailed ultrasound should be arranged to check fetal growth, quantify the amniotic fluid index and examine for fetal abnormality. (1 mark)

Fetal abnormalities that can cause polyhydramnios include the following:

- Neuromuscular conditions that have the effect of obstructing the swallowing of amniotic fluid by the fetus.
- Fetal gastrointestinal abnormalities, including oesophageal and duodenal atresia. These block the ingestions of liquor into the fetus.
- Fetal hydrops, which should be excluded on an ultrasound scan, as this is associated with polyhydramnios secondary to cardiac failure or anaemia.
- Twin-to-twin transfusion is a rare cause of acute polyhydramnios in the recipient sac of monochorionic twins. It is associated with oligohydramnios in the other sac and requires urgent treatment by amniodrainage. (4 marks)
- A detailed examination of the placenta may reveal a chorioangioma. (1 mark)

See Chapter 8, *Obstetrics by Ten Teachers*, 19th edition.

Twins and higher order multiple gestations

9 Outline the complications that may occur with a twin pregnancy.
Complications that occur in twins can be divided into those that occur in all twins and those that occur specifically in monochorionic twins. Monochorionic twins have specific complications owing to the fact that the twins share the same placenta. (2 marks)

The overall perinatal mortality rate for twins is six times higher than for singletons. The main contributing factor to this high rate is preterm delivery. (2 marks)

Spontaneous preterm delivery is an ever-present risk in any twin pregnancy and approximately half of all twin pregnancies deliver prematurely. Uterine over-distension is thought to be the primary reason for preterm labour in twins. In a dichorionic pregnancy, the chance of late miscarriage is approximately 2 per cent, and for mono-chorionic twins the risk is as high as 12 per cent. (2 marks)

Compared with singleton pregnancies, the risk of poor growth is higher in each individual twin alone and substantially raised in the pregnancy as a whole. In dichorionic twins, each fetus runs twice the risk of a low birthweight and there is a 20 per cent chance that at least one twin will suffer poor growth. The chance of poor fetal growth for monochorionic twins is almost double that for dichorionic twins. (3 marks)

Compared with singleton pregnancies, twins carry at least twice the risk of a baby with a birth defect. Each dichorionic twin pregnancy has at least twice the risk of a structural anomaly. In contrast, monochorionic twins carry a risk that is four times higher. (2 marks)

Chromosomal abnormality risk increases with maternal age independent of the number of fetuses. Therefore, in monozygotic twins, the risk is the same as for maternal age as both fetuses arise from the same egg. However, dizygotic twins have twice the risk, as the fetuses come from two different eggs. (2 marks)

All monochorionic twins share vascular anastomoses and it is an imbalance in the blood flow across these anastomoses that causes the specific complication of twin–twin transfusion syndrome. Monoamniotic twins have the additional risk of cord entanglement, causing fetal death late in pregnancy. (2 marks)

The larger placental area formed in twin pregnancies gives a higher risk of pre-eclampsia. Twin pregnancy may also be associated with assisted conception, which gives a higher risk of preterm delivery. (2 marks)

See Chapter 9, *Obstetrics by Ten Teachers*, 19th edition.

Pre-eclampsia and other disorders of placentation

10 A twenty four-year-old woman presents at 36 weeks in her first pregnancy. She has a blood pressure of 140/100 mmHg and urine dipstix shows 3+ proteinuria. Outline the management of this woman.
The most likely diagnosis is pre-eclampsia; however, this needs to be confirmed. A full history is required to ascertain whether there are any risk factors for pre-eclampsia. These include a family history of pre-eclampsia and multiple pregnancy. A detailed history of symptoms should be taken, particularly of headache, visual disturbance and epigastric pain. (2 marks)

A full medical examination of the woman should be undertaken, including a neurological examination of reflexes, which are brisk in pre-eclampsia. Clonus should be specifically sought and fundoscopy performed. An abdominal palpation will demonstrate whether the fetus is clinically small for dates. (3 marks)

The woman should be admitted for both maternal and fetal assessment. Maternal assessment should include a full blood count to determine platelet count. Urea and electrolytes should be determined to assess renal function. Serum uric acid levels should also be measured as these reflect both renal function and placental breakdown. Liver function tests should also be performed. A 24-hour urine collection should be initiated to confirm that the urinary protein is >0.3g/24 hours. An urgent mid-stream urine and microscopy should be sent to exclude a urinary tract infection. (3 marks)

Cardiotocography should be performed to assess immediate fetal well-being. If there are any abnormalities noted, then delivery should be considered. An ultrasound scan is useful to determine fetal well-being and presentation. (2 marks)

Delivery should be considered in this scenario. A vaginal examination should be performed to assess whether the cervix is favourable. If the cervix is unfavourable, then induction with prostaglandin pessaries is indicated.

If an artificial rupture of the membranes is possible, this should be undertaken. The fetus should be monitored continuously throughout labour. This woman requires close observation with regard to blood pressure and urine output, and one-to-one midwifery care.   (3 marks)

See Chapter 10, *Obstetrics by Ten Teachers*, 19th edition.

Late miscarriage and early birth

11 Define second trimester miscarriage and outline the possible aetiologies.
Second trimester miscarriage is defined as a pregnancy loss occurring between 12 and 23 weeks' gestation.
                                                                                             (1 mark)

The likely aetiologies behind second trimester losses vary with gestation. At 12–16 weeks, the predominant cause will be the same as first trimester losses: fetal chromosomal and structural anomalies. A more practical definition of late miscarriage is one occurring between 17 and 23 weeks.   (2 marks)

A specific iatrogenic risk factor for late miscarriage is mid-trimester amniocentesis. This is usually performed at between 16 and 18 weeks' gestation and carries a risk of miscarriage of 1 in 200.   (2 marks)

At the end of the second trimester, between 19 and 23 weeks, the most common factors underlying miscarriage will be those linked to premature labour. Over-distension of the uterus, either by multiple pregnancy or polyhydramnios, leads to increased myometrial contractility and premature shortening and opening of the cervix.
                                                                                             (4 marks)

Intrauterine bleeding, for example from a subchorional haematoma, irritates the uterus, leading to contractions, membrane damage and early rupture.   (1 mark)

Ascending infection from the vagina may pass through the cervix and reach the fetal membranes. This may have the effect of stimulating prostaglandin release and trigger contraction of the uterus.   (2 marks)

Cervical weakness that has occurred as a result of previous surgical injury or a congenital defect may allow the cervix to shorten and open prematurely; the membranes then prolapse and may be damaged by stretching or direct contact with a bacterial pathogen.   (2 marks)

See Chapter 11, *Obstetrics by Ten Teachers*, 19th edition.

Preterm labour

12 A twenty seven-year-old woman, who is at 30 weeks' gestation in her first pregnancy, is admitted from home with a history of painful contractions. Outline the management of this problem.
The most important diagnosis to exclude in the scenario is that of preterm labour with or without membrane rupture.   (1 mark)

The first step is to take the relevant history. This should determine whether there are any risk factors for either preterm labour or preterm rupture of the membranes (PROM). The common risk factors for both PROM and preterm labour that should be enquired about are twin pregnancy, uterine abnormalities and cervical damage (cone biopsy or repeat dilatation). It should also be determined whether there is a history of recurrent antepartum haemorrhage or sepsis. A full social history should be taken to determine whether the woman smokes or takes drugs, and her social class, as all these factors increase the risk of preterm labour.
                                                                                             (4 marks)

The diagnosis of preterm labour is difficult as women often present with vague cramp-like pains and discomfort. The coexistence of bleeding should always be taken seriously. An increased analgesia requirement can also help refine the diagnosis. The most reliable diagnostic feature of PROM from the history is that of a sudden rush of fluid per vaginum. (3 marks)

A full examination should be undertaken. Abdominal palpation may reveal the presence of uterine tenderness, suggesting abruption or chorioamnionitis. Infection may lead to an increased pulse and temperature. A careful speculum examination should be performed to determine whether there is any pooling of liquor and a visual assessment of cervical dilatation is possible. While the speculum examination is being undertaken, a high vaginal swab (HVS), a fetal fibronectin swab and a nitrazine test can be performed. A negative fibronectin test gives a low chance of delivery within the subsequent 2 weeks. Similarly a positive nitrazine test increases the probability of PROM. (2 marks)

Maternal well-being should be assessed with measurement of blood pressure, pulse and temperature. A full blood count should be performed to determine whether there is an increase in the white-cell count, indicating infection. A mid-stream specimen of urine should be sent for culture and microscopy, as the symptoms of urinary infection may mimic those of preterm labour. (3 marks)

Fetal assessment should include CTG to determine whether there is a fetal tachycardia indicative of infection. An ultrasound scan can yield important information on liquor volume and cervical length can be determined if PROM has been excluded. (2 marks)

Maternal steroids should be given to induce fetal lung maturity. Tocolysis should be considered to allow the administration of maternal steroids. If PROM has been confirmed, then a 10-day course of erythromycin should be commenced, as this has been shown to improve neonatal outcome. If the HVS is positive for beta-haemolytic streptococcus, intravenous antibiotics should be administered during labour. If labour continues, continuous fetal monitoring should be initiated. (3 marks)

See Chapter 11, *Obstetrics by Ten Teachers*, 18th edition.

Medical diseases complicating pregnancy

13 **A twenty four-year-old woman with poorly controlled insulin-dependent diabetes attends a GP clinic. She is planning to start a family. Outline the advice specific to her condition that you would give regarding pregnancy.**
The woman should be advised that poor glucose control in pregnancy increases the risk of congenital anomalies and also increases the risk of miscarriage. However, with good control, these risks are substantially reduced. Target HbA1c prior to conception should be <6.5 per cent. (2 marks)

She will require hospital care and this will take the form of a joint clinic with an obstetrician, diabetic physician, diabetic nurses and dieticians. She should be advised to take high-dose folic acid (5 mg) pre-conception and for the first 12 weeks of the pregnancy. (2 marks)

The aim of treatment is to maintain the blood glucose levels as near normal as possible. Insulin requirements go up during pregnancy and these will need careful monitoring. The woman should monitor her own blood glucose levels and have blood taken for HbA1c to monitor long-term control. She is at increased risk of both diabetic ketoacidosis and hypoglycaemia, and should be educated about the signs and symptoms of both. (3 marks)

It should be explained that an ultrasound scan at approximately 20 weeks' gestation would examine for structural anomalies, especially cardiac and neural tube defects. (2 marks)

There is also a risk that both diabetic nephropathy and retinopathy will worsen with pregnancy; however, these complications usually improve post-delivery. There is an increased risk of pre-eclampsia, which will require regular monitoring of blood pressure and urine. (2 marks)

There is also an increased risk of polyhydramnios, which is associated with an increase in premature delivery. Poor glycaemic control is associated with macrosomia and an increased rate of shoulder dystocia. Careful fetal monitoring will be necessary and induction of labour is considered after 38/40 due to the increased unexplained stillbirth rate. (4 marks)

During labour, normoglycaemia should be maintained using a sliding scale of insulin and blood glucose should be tested hourly. Continuous fetal monitoring will be required during labour in view of the increased risk of this pregnancy. (2 marks)

See Chapter 12, *Obstetrics by Ten Teachers*, 19th edition.

Perinatal infections

14 Write short notes on HIV, parvovirus and Group B streptococcus in pregnancy.

HIV
This is caused by an RNA retrovirus. There is no indication that pregnancy causes the progression of the disease in the mother. There is no evidence that pregnancy increases the risk of progression from HIV to the acquired immunodeficiency syndrome (AIDS). (3 marks)

HIV has been shown to have specific effects on the pregnancy; there is an increased risk of miscarriage, preterm delivery and intrauterine growth restriction. Caregivers should maintain confidentiality during pregnancy and delivery. (3 marks)

Vertical transmission occurs in 25–40 per cent of pregnancies where there is no intervention. It is thought that the majority of transmission occurs around the time of delivery and subsequent breastfeeding. Three interventions have been shown to reduce the vertical transmission rate: avoiding breastfeeding, elective Caesarean section (where the viral load is >50 copies/mL), and antiviral medication during the later half of pregnancy and into the neonatal period. (4 marks)

Parvovirus
Parvovirus B19 is the cause of slapped cheek syndrome in children. The infection is asymptomatic in 50 per cent of children and 25 per cent of adults. (2 marks)

In approximately 15 per cent of infections occurring during pregnancy, the fetus becomes chronically infected. This leads to a persistent anaemia *in utero*, which may develop into non-immune hydrops. This may resolve spontaneously or may require a blood transfusion. (3 marks)

The diagnosis of primary parvovirus is confirmed by demonstration of virus-specific IgM in the maternal serum. If this is demonstrated within the maternal serum, then the fetus needs close monitoring for signs of hydrops. However, parvovirus is not a teratogenic virus. (3 marks)

Group B streptococcus
This is an asymptomatic bacterial commensal of the gut and genital tract. It is carried asymptomatically in approximately 20–40 per cent of women. (2 marks)

It may cause severe neonatal infection and death. Although it can be detected on vaginal culture, screening and treatment are not beneficial because of frequent recolonization post-treatment. (2 marks)

Therefore, the recommendation is that the organism should be sought by culture in complicated pregnancies or where there has been a previous preterm delivery. (2 marks)

The infants most at risk are premature, those with prolonged rupture of membranes and growth-restricted fetuses. (2 marks)

There is no good evidence to support the use of intrapartum antibiotic prophylaxis in women who have had Group B streptococcus carriage in a previous pregnancy.   (1 mark)

See Chapter 13, *Obstetrics by Ten Teachers*, 19th edition.

Labour

15 Define primary dysfunctional labour, and outline its causes and possible treatments.
Primary dysfunctional labour is defined as poor progress, normal progress being >1 cm per hour of cervical dilatation in the active phase of labour. However, progress is considered abnormal only if it occurs at <1 cm every 2 hours.   (2 marks)

The progress of labour depends on three interconnected variables: the powers, the passages and the passenger.   (2 marks)

The most common cause of poor progress is ineffective uterine action, which is more common in the primiparous woman. The treatment modalities that are available are rehydration, artificial rupture of the fetal membranes and intravenous synthetic oxytocin.   (2 marks)

For adequate progress in labour, the tight application of the presenting part to the cervix is vital. Therefore, any malpresentations of the passenger, such as a brow or breech presentation, may ultimately result in slow progress.   (2 marks)

Cephalopelvic disproportion (CPD) is also a cause of primary dysfunctional labour and implies anatomical disproportion between the fetal head and the pelvis. It can be due to a large head, a small pelvis or a combination of both. It should be suspected if labour progresses slowly despite oxytocin, the fetal head fails to engage, vaginal examination shows severe moulding and caput, and the head is poorly applied to the cervix. Oxytocin may overcome the relative CPD of an abnormal presentation, such as brow, but Caesarean section may be the only recourse if the fetus is in an unfavourable position.   (3 marks)

Although abnormalities of the bony pelvis may cause delay of labour, abnormalities of the uterus and the cervix may have a similar effect. An unsuspected lower uterine fibroid can delay descent of the fetal head and result in Caesarean section. Cervical dystocia, owing to a scarred non-compliant cervix, can also result in a similar outcome.   (3 marks)

See Chapter 14, *Obstetrics by Ten Teachers*, 19th edition.

Operative interventions in obstetrics

16 Write short notes on ventouse and forceps.

Ventouse
This is an instrument that uses suction to aid the delivery of the fetus. It can be used for both maternal and fetal indications. The main maternal indication is exhaustion after prolonged pushing in the second stage, but it may also be used when shortening of the second stage is an advantage, such as with maternal cardiac disease. The main fetal indication is suspected fetal compromise in the second stage.   (4 marks)

The contraindications to its use are face presentation, gestation < 35 weeks and marked bleeding from a fetal blood sample site. The prerequisites for delivery with the ventouse are a fully dilated cervix, station of the fetal head below the ischial spines, position known, good contractions, maternal bladder empty, adequate analgesia and maternal co-operation.   (6 marks)

The most common maternal complication is genital tract trauma. The main fetal complications are cephalo-haematoma and, rarely, serious intracranial injuries. (2 marks)

Forceps
Obstetric forceps can be divided into two distinct groups: non-rotational or rotational forceps. (2 marks)

Non-rotational forceps have similar maternal and fetal indications to the ventouse. Non-rotational forceps have both a cephalic and a pelvic curve. Although the general indications for forceps and ventouse are similar, there are several specific indications for forceps: face presentation, bleeding from a fetal blood sample, the after-coming head of a breech presentation, and delivery prior to 35 completed weeks. Obstetric forceps can also be used to aid delivery of the fetal head at Caesarean section. (6 marks)

Kielland's (rotational) forceps lack the pelvic curve and this allows their rotation within the pelvis. The rotational forceps have additional indications for malpresentations, such as an occipital posterior position or deep transverse arrest. (2 marks)

The most common maternal complication is maternal trauma. The forceps are less likely to cause cephalo-haematoma but may cause rare, serious, intracranial injuries or facial nerve palsies. (2 marks)

See Chapter 15, *Obstetrics by Ten Teachers*, 19th edition.

Obstetric emergencies

17 Write short notes on cord prolapse, shoulder dystocia and primary postpartum haemorrhage.

Cord prolapse
This is defined as a loop or loops of umbilical cord that fall through the cervix in front of the presenting part. Cord prolapse is associated with prematurity and malpresentations. This occurs in approximately 1 in 500 deliveries. (2 marks)

The diagnosis is usually made on vaginal examination because of an abnormal CTG. If the cord is through the vulva, it should be replaced to keep it warm. Urgent Caesarean section is required unless the cervix is fully dilated and assisted delivery can be performed safely. (4 marks)

While the Caesarean section is being arranged, it is vital that the pressure on the umbilical vein is reduced to allow oxygen to pass to the fetus. This is achieved by placing the mother on all fours in a 'head down' position. A hand should be placed in the vagina to push the presenting part up. Filling the bladder may help to elevate the presenting part and relieve pressure on the cord. (2 marks)

Outcome depends on many factors, including gestation and other pregnancy complications. (1 mark)

Shoulder dystocia
This is defined as difficulty in delivery of the anterior fetal shoulder. The incidence varies between 0.2 per cent and 1.2 per cent of deliveries. (2 marks)

There are several risk factors that predispose to shoulder dystocia. These are large fetus, small mother, maternal obesity, diabetes mellitus, prolonged first stage of labour, prolonged second stage of labour and assisted vaginal delivery. (2 marks)

Shoulder dystocia should be managed by a sequence of manoeuvres designed to facilitate delivery without fetal damage. The initial response to a shoulder dystocia should be a call for senior help. Excess traction should be avoided at all times. McRobert's manoeuvre is employed, where the maternal legs are hyperflexed and abducted at the hips. Suprapubic pressure should be applied to adduct the fetal shoulders. This should overcome 85 percent of shoulder dystocia. If this fails, more complex manoeuvres are required. These involve internal rotation of the fetal shoulders and delivery of the posterior arm.   (4 marks)

Following delivery, the mother and her partner need to be debriefed regarding the events surrounding the delivery.   (2 marks)

Postpartum haemorrhage
This is defined as excess blood loss (500 mL) after delivery. This can be further subdivided into primary (within the first 24 hours) and secondary (up to 6 weeks) postpartum haemorrhage.   (2 marks)

The first step in management is maternal resuscitation, with facial oxygen, intravenous access and fluids. Blood should be sent for full blood count and urgent cross-match.   (1 mark)

The most common cause of massive blood loss is uterine atony. This accounts for 90 per cent of cases. The first step is to stop the bleeding, which can be initially achieved by uterine massage or bimanual compression. Uterine contraction can then be maintained by pharmacological methods; these include the use of ergometrine and high-dose Syntocinon. The bladder should be emptied to aid contraction. If the uterus still fails to respond, prostaglandin F2-alpha can be administered systemically or directly into the myometrium.   (4 marks)

If the placenta has not been delivered, this should be expedited. The placenta and membranes should be checked for completeness, as retained tissue is a major cause of postpartum haemorrhage.   (1 mark)

However, if the bleeding continues despite adequate uterine contraction, the next most common cause is genital tract trauma. The patient will require an examination under anaesthesia to explore the genital tract and repair the damage sustained.   (2 marks)

If bleeding still persists, then clotting should be checked urgently as disseminated vascular coagulation may be present and needs to be corrected with blood products.   (2 marks)

See Chapter 16, *Obstetrics by Ten Teachers*, 19th edition.

The puerperium

18 A twenty six-year-old woman who is 8 days post normal delivery is admitted pyrexial at 38.5°C. Discuss the possible diagnoses, investigations and treatments.
Postpartum pyrexia is a relatively common occurrence, with an incidence of approximately 5 per cent. The aetiology can be broadly divided into three separate categories: infection of the urogenital tract, breast engorgement/infective mastalgia, and distant infection.   (3 marks)

The most common cause of post-natal pyrexia is a urinary tract infection. The patient will present with dysuria, frequency and lower abdominal pain. This pain will be localized over the bladder and may radiate to the loins. A clean-catch urine specimen should be collected and dipstick analysis may show protein and nitrates. The specimen should be sent for microscopy and culture. A full blood count and urea and electrolytes should be sent as a general investigation of all women with pyrexia. Antibiotic therapy should be initiated; however, this should be altered depending on the results of the urine culture.   (5 marks)

Endometritis is another common infection that may occur in the post-natal period. It presents with fever, rigors and an associated offensive vaginal discharge. A vaginal swab should be taken and antibiotics commenced. The possibility of retained products of conception should be considered.   (3 marks)

Breast engorgement/infective mastalgia will present with a history of breast pain. Examination may reveal an enlarged erythematous breast. Anti-inflammatory drugs can be used to alleviate the pain, along with antibiotics if infection is considered. If a breast abscess is present, it will need incision and drainage.   (4 marks)

Chest infections are another cause of pyrexia that needs to be excluded, especially in a patient with an underlying chest problem, such as asthma. The patient may present with a productive cough. Examination would reveal evidence of consolidation at the lung bases. Sputum should be sent for culture. Antibiotics and supportive therapy with oxygen and physiotherapy are required.   (3 marks)

Deep vein thrombosis (DVT) may present as a postpartum pyrexia. The patient may complain of a painful swollen leg and calf tenderness. Examination would reveal an enlarged calf that would be red, swollen and hot to the touch. A duplex Doppler of the leg would confirm the diagnosis. Anticoagulant treatment should be initiated.   (3 marks)

A pulmonary embolism may also present with pyrexia and therefore any patient where the diagnosis is questioned should be investigated. This may necessitate a ventilation/perfusion (V/Q) scan and treatment with anticoagulants.   (2 marks)

See Chapter 17, *Obstetrics by Ten Teachers*, 19th edition.

Psychiatric disorders in pregnancy and the puerperium

19 Discuss the possible psychiatric sequelae of pregnancy and how they might be treated.
Disturbances in the emotional state are common in the post-natal period. Up to 80 per cent of women will experience some form of emotional alteration. It most commonly occurs between days 3 and 10.   (2 marks)

Mild post-natal depression affects 7 per cent of women. It is associated with social adversity, single status and poor support. The history is an insidious onset of insomnia and difficulty in coping. The most effective treatment for mild depression is counselling, which in this group is as effective as antidepressant therapy. (4 marks)

Severe post-natal depression occurs in 3–5 per cent of all women. Most cases can be detected at the 6-week post-natal check by use of the Edinburgh post-natal score. A total of 30 per cent of those women with this condition will present within the first three months after delivery. They may present with a history of early morning wakening, altered appetite and ahedonism. Management should include explanation and reassurance. Tricyclic antidepressant therapy is effective, with results observed within 2 weeks of commencing treatment. Selective serotonin reuptake inhibitors (SSRIs) are also used, although the evidence for safety in breastfeeding is less well established. The course should be maintained for six months.   (4 marks)

Postpartum psychosis affects 2 in 1000 women. One-third of these women will present will an acute episode of mania, while the other two-thirds will present with depression. Acute management should be aimed at sedation with neuroleptic drugs, which allows both containment and assessment.   (3 marks)

A psychiatrist with an interest in postpartum psychiatric disorders should perform an assessment and it should coincide with admission to the nearest mother and baby unit. The patient should be continued on an oral neuroleptic agent, such as haloperidol. However, these drugs have extrapyramidal side effects, which can be treated with procyclidine. Lithium carbonate can be used for the mother who presents with a manic pathology. For women with severe depression, electroconvulsive therapy can be used as a first-line treatment. The mother should be continued on treatment for at least six months and advised that there is a 50 per cent recurrence rate.   (3 marks)

See Chapter 18, *Obstetrics by Ten Teachers*, 19th edition.

Neonatology

20 Describe the checks that should be undertaken on newborn babies prior to leaving hospital.
A physical examination of every neonate is a core part of the UK child health surveillance programme. The examination should be carried out within 72 hours of birth and aims to identify major and minor congenital

abnormalities. There is also an important role in continuing health screening, education and parental reassurance. (3 marks)

The examiner should acquaint themselves with the antenatal and birth history. The family history may be relevant, for example in developmental dysplasia of the hip. Any parental concerns should be carefully addressed. (2 marks)

The baby should be undressed apart from the nappy and a general inspection undertaken, including skin, colour and any dysmorphic features of the face or neck. The scalp and fontanelles should be gently palpated and head circumference measured. The palate should be gently assessed with a finger in the infant's mouth. (3 marks)

The heart rate and respiratory rate should be counted. The heart sounds should be listened to and any murmurs identified. The abdomen should be gently palpated for masses. The red reflex should be elicited bilaterally with an ophthalmoscope. (3 marks)

The nappy should then be cautiously removed and the femoral pulses felt. An inspection of the external genitalia and anus should be carried out. (2 marks)

The infant should be turned prone to inspect the spine. This provides a good opportunity to assess tone. Other primitive reflexes should be checked for, including the rooting reflex and the startle reflex. (2 marks)

Finally, testing for hip dislocation should be performed. The parents should be given a brief summary of the findings and any follow-up required, with appropriate reassurance and explanation. (2 marks)

See Chapter 19, *Obstetrics by Ten Teachers*, 19th edition.

Ethical and medicolegal issues in obstetric practice

21 **A twenty four-year old woman in spontaneous labour at 38 weeks with her first baby has a sudden prolonged fetal bradycardia on CTG. You wish to prepare her for an emergency Caesarean section. What steps do you need to take to ensure her consent to the operation is valid?**

Valid consent must be obtained prior to starting the procedure; to do otherwise is an assault on the woman. In law, a competent adult retains the right to make decisions and refuse treatment, even if these decisions appear unwise. Ideally, her consent will be recorded in written form, with a record of all the risks and benefits that have been discussed with her. Her informed consent to the procedure is still valid, however, even if not in written form. If the woman withholds her consent to a procedure that is thought to be in her best interests by the obstetric team, then she should be fully counselled regarding the risks of not proceeding. If she still refuses to undergo the procedure, her decision should be respected and all discussions fully documented. (4 marks)

The woman must be able to understand the information given, and steps should be taken to maximize her understanding, for example providing translation if required. No one can give consent on behalf of another adult in UK law, so the woman must be given every opportunity to understand the information, including analgesia as necessary. (2 marks)

The woman must be able to weigh the information given, which may be difficult in the extremely stressful situation of an emergency Caesarean section. Although time may be critical, she should have information regarding the risks and benefits to enable her to come to an informed choice. (2 marks)

Informed consent is further dependent on the woman being able to communicate her choice to the medical team. After consenting to the procedure she retains the right to change her mind and withdraw consent at any time. (2 marks)

If the woman is felt to lack capacity, for example due to a pre-existing condition, then the law empowers medical professionals to act in her best interests. (1 mark)

See Chapter 20, *Obstetrics by Ten Teachers*, 19th edition.

OBJECTIVE STRUCTURED CLINICAL EXAMINATION QUESTIONS

QUESTIONS

1 Physiological changes in pregnancy

A twenty five-year-old woman in her first pregnancy attends booking clinic at 12 weeks' gestation.

a) Describe the cardiovascular changes that have occurred.
b) Outline the physiological function and changes that have occurred in human chorionic gonadotrophin.

This lady goes on to have a normal vaginal delivery at term. She opts to breastfeed the baby.

c) Outline the physiological changes that occur within the mother with breastfeeding.

2 Normal fetal development

A twenty two-year-old is admitted to the labour ward at 27 weeks' pregnant. She is complaining of regular painful tightening. She describes having a mucus show the previous night, but denies any history of preterm rupture of membranes. On examination she is distressed and requiring analgesia. Vaginal examination reveals that she is fully dilated with bulging forewaters. She delivers a live female infant that weighs 800 g.

a) Describe the physiological changes that occur in the cardiovascular circulation with birth.
b) Describe the physiological changes that occur in the respiratory system with birth.
c) What are the four main risks to the baby of premature delivery and how can these be minimized?

3 Antenatal care

A thirty-year-old woman attends a routine booking clinic.

a) What are the key elements of a booking history?
b) Explain the tests and scans that the woman will have during pregnancy, assuming she has no risk factors.

4 Antenatal imaging and fetal assessment

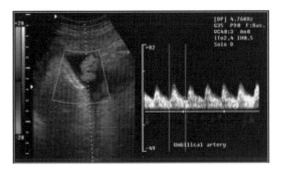

a) What is this investigation?
b) What is this picture showing?
c) What is RI?
d) What waveforms are abnormal?
e) What does it predict?

5 Prenatal diagnosis

A couple arrive in your antenatal clinic. They are both known to be carriers of the common mutation of cystic fibrosis.

a) What are the chances of having a baby affected by cystic fibrosis?
b) What is the most common mutation of the gene?
c) How can the diagnosis be made prenatally?
d) How early may the prenatal diagnostic test be made?

6 Second trimester miscarriage

Miss M is a 22-year-old single parent. She has had two previous miscarriages from two different partners. Her last pregnancy ended in a miscarriage at 18 weeks after she was admitted with backache. She is now 22 weeks' pregnant by her dating scan. She has been admitted to the labour ward with low back pain and a mucus loss.

a) What is the likely diagnosis?
b) What are the key points in the examination and investigation?

Miss M then starts to have painful regular contractions.

c) How would you manage her labour?

7 Antenatal obstetric complications

The community midwife refers a twenty five-year-old woman in her second pregnancy to the antenatal clinic. Clinical examination has shown the fetus to be in the breech position. An ultrasound scan confirms an extended breech presentation. You are asked to counsel this lady as to the possible options that are available for her management.

8 Twins and higher-order multiple gestations

A thirty two-year-old woman attends your booking clinic. She has just had a dating scan that confirms the presence of twins. The ultrasound report demonstrates that these are monochorionic diamniotic twins.

a) Define monozygotic twins.
b) Describe how chorionicity is determined by ultrasound scan.
c) Outline the risk of multiple pregnancy.
d) Outline the specific risks of monochorionic twins.

9 Disorders of placentation

An eighteen-year-old woman in her first pregnancy is admitted to the antenatal ward for observation. She is 26 weeks pregnant. Consider the following blood results:

Table 5.1		
	24 weeks	**26 weeks**
Serum urate	150 μmol/L	230 μmol/L
24-hour urinary protein	0.6 g/hours	3.5 g/hours
Platelet count	230	120

a) What is the most likely diagnosis?
b) List three maternal signs that would help guide our management.
c) What are three possible maternal complications of this disease if it remains untreated?
d) What investigations would you perform on the fetus?
e) How should this woman be managed?

10 Preterm labour

A twenty six-year-old Caucasian woman presented at 25 weeks' gestation in her first pregnancy. She gave a good history of ruptured membranes 3 hours prior to admission. On clinical examination no uterine activity was noted. The maternal blood pressure was 140/75 mmHg, the temperature was 37⁰C and the pulse rate was 80 beats per minute. An aseptic speculum examination revealed clear fluid in the vagina.

a) Outline four investigations that would be useful in the further management of this patient with confirmed ruptured fetal membranes.
b) At what gestational age can a fetus survive outside the womb?

c) With regard to women delivering after preterm rupture of the fetal membranes, what post-natal complications are important?

d) How would you advise this woman in her next pregnancy?

11 Medical diseases of pregnancy

Mrs MV is known to have pre-existing cardiac disease.

a) What is the most common acquired cardiac lesion?
b) What are the effects of cardiac disease on pregnancy?
c) How should her labour be managed?

12 Perinatal infections

A thirty five-year-old woman comes to the booking clinic. She has had a routine HIV test at her booking visit, which has shown her to be HIV positive. She has been counselled regarding the diagnosis of HIV.

a) What type of virus is HIV?
b) Name two types of cell that have CD4 receptors.
c) Outline two strategies of treatment that are available.
d) What interventions have been shown to reduce the transmission of HIV to the baby?

13 Labour

Instructions to candidates:

You are asked to examine the chart.

Name:		
Affix Identity Label	Date 30-08-2002 Parity 0	Special Instructions
	EDD 01-09-2002 Blood Group Rh+Ve	
D.O.B: 07-01-79		

Membranes Ruptured		Spontaneous Show First Noted	Date: 29-08-02	Onset of Labour Contractions
Amniotomy	Date		Date: 30-08-02	
Spontaneous	Time		Time: 00.30	Time: 06.00

a) What is the chart called?
b) Describe the chart in front of you.
c) Describe the stages of labour.
d) What abnormal labour pattern does the diagram illustrate?
e) How would you manage this obstetric problem?

14 Operative interventions in obstetrics

The illustration shows an instrument that will be seen on any labour ward.

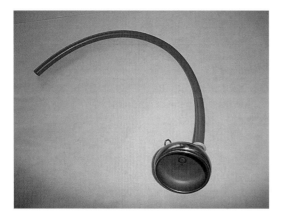

a) Name the instrument in the picture.
b) Give three indications for its use.
c) Give three situations where this instrument is contraindicated.
d) Give two maternal complications of this instrument.
e) What are the possible fetal complications of this instrument?

15 Obstetric emergencies

Mrs Smith has delivered a 3500 g baby at the delivery suite. Mrs Smith was given intramuscular syntometrine. However, she has continued to lose blood and the estimate is 1000 mL. She is not clinically shocked and you are to see her because of her blood loss.

a) Define postpartum haemorrhage.
b) List the action you would take once you arrived to see this patient.
c) List the four most common causes of postpartum haemorrhage.

16 The puerperium

You are asked to see a thirty seven-year-old woman on the labour ward. She had an emergency Caesarean section for breech presentation 8 days ago. Over the last few hours she has become breathless and has developed chest pain.

a) What is the most likely diagnosis?
b) What in the history would you ask to aid your diagnosis?
c) What would you look for on examination?
d) What investigations would you carry out to confirm the diagnosis?
e) What are the treatment options?

17 Psychiatric disorders in pregnancy and the puerperium

A twenty seven-year-old mother is seen by the community midwife 5 weeks after having a Caesarean section for failure to progress in the first stage of labour. She describes being miserable and starts to cry.

a) What is the mostly likely diagnosis?
b) What other symptoms might she have?
c) How is this condition treated?
d) Name a psychiatric disorder specific to pregnancy.
e) Outline the treatments that are available.

18 Neonatology

a) List three different deliveries where a trained neonatal resuscitator should be present.
b) Describe the Apgar score and how it is used.
c) Describe how you would manage a neonate who has been delivered without respiratory effort but with a heart rate of >100 bpm and who is centrally cyanosed.
d) Describe level 2 neonatal intensive care.

1 Physiological changes in pregnancy

a) Pregnancy is associated with dramatic cardiovascular changes, which occur from an early gestation. Overall there is a 10–20 per cent increase in the maternal heart rate and 10 per cent increase in the stroke volume. These increase the cardiac output by 30–50 per cent. Associated with these changes are decreases in the maternal mean arterial pressure and in the peripheral vascular resistance.

b) Human chorionic gonadotrophin is composed of α and β subunits. HCG levels increase dramatically over the first 10 weeks. After 10 weeks HCG reduces in concentration until 12 weeks when it plateaus for the remainder of pregnancy. During early pregnancy HCG has a major role in maintaining the function of the corpus luteum and the production of progesterone.

c) The serum prolactin concentrations increase throughout pregnancy. However, it does not promote lactation during this time as its function is antagonized by oestrogen. The rapid fall in oestrogen within the first 48 hours after birth allow lactation to occur. Early sucking promotes lactation by increasing the posterior pituitary release of oxytocin and prolactin. Oxytocin causes the myoepithelial cells to contract and express milk, and prolactin increases milk synthesis.

See Chapter 3, *Obstetrics by Ten Teachers,* 19th edition.

2 Normal fetal development

a) At birth the cardiovascular system undergoes extensive remodelling under the changed haemodynamics of the now activated pulmonary system. In addition, the cessation of the umbilical blood flow in the ductus venosus causes a fall in the right atrial pressure and closure of the foramen ovale. Ventilation of the lungs opens the pulmonary circulation, with a rapid fall in the pulmonary vasculature. The ductus arteriosus closes functionally within a few days of birth.

b) The fluid within the lung is reabsorbed. Compression of the chest at delivery forces out approximately one third of the fluid, and the release of adrenalin promotes reabsorption of the rest. Surfactant is released, triggered by adrenalin and steroids. There is a fall in the capillary pressure of the lungs that occurs with the expansion of the alveoli, and the vasodilatory effect of oxygen. Respiratory movements of the chest commence.

c) Respiratory distress syndrome may lead to hypoxia. The administration of antenatal steroids to the mother reduces the risk and severity. In this case antenatal steroids were not administered; however, the severity of respiratory distress syndrome can be reduced by the administration of surfactant. Hypothermia is a common problem related to the large surface area, lack of subcutaneous fat and keratinized skin. This large surface area also predisposes to dehydration. This can be reduced by nursing the infant in an incubator. Jaundice secondary to liver immaturity is common in the preterm infant. This can be treated with phototherapy. Periventricular haemorrhage and intraventricular haemorrhage commonly lead to cerebral palsy.

See Chapter 4, *Obstetrics by Ten Teachers,* 19th edition.

3 Antenatal care

a) The booking history should include:
Name
Age
Occupation

Obstetric history
Medical history
Treatment history
Social history

b) This question is best approached by dividing it into tests that are performed during the various trimesters of pregnancy.

First trimester:

All pregnant women are encouraged to undergo screening for a number of health issues, which may have an impact on the pregnancy or the fetus. The following tests are performed routinely during the first trimesters:

- A full blood count is used to screen for anaemia and thrombocytopenia, both of which may require further investigation.
- Maternal blood group is determined, which will help with cross-matching at a later date. Rhesus status will be determined and prophylaxis will be offered at 28 and 34 weeks if the mother is Rhesus negative.
- Rubella status will be determined as vertical transmission carries serious risk of congenital abnormalities, especially in the first trimester. Women who are found to be non-immune should be advised to avoid infectious contacts.
- Hepatitis B status should be determined, so that passive and active immunization can be offered to baby post delivery.
- All women should be offered HIV testing as the use of antiretroviral agents, elective Caesarean section and avoidance of breastfeeding reduce the vertical transmission to less than 5 per cent.
- A dating ultrasound would be offered to all women. This has the benefit of accurate dating.

Second trimester:

During the second trimester at around 15 weeks the triple test is offered to all pregnant women. This is used to advise the mother of her risk of having a baby with Down's syndrome.

Third trimester:

Measurement of blood pressure occurs at all antenatal visits; however, its main role is during the late second and early third trimester as a screening test for pre-eclampsia.

Urine will be analysed at all antenatal visits for protein, blood and glucose. This is used to detect infection, pre-eclampsia and gestational diabetes.

See Chapter 5, *Obstetrics by Ten Teachers,* 19th edition.

4 Antenatal imaging and fetal assessment

a) This is an umbilical artery Doppler.
b) The picture shows a normal umbilical artery Doppler waveform.
c) Resistive Index. This is calculated from maximum umbilical artery systolic velocity – minimum umbilical end diastolic velocity/maximum umbilical artery systolic velocity. When this value rises above the 95th centile of the range, this implies that the fetal placental perfusion is faulty.
d) Absent or reversed end diastolic flow.
e) Absent or reversed end diastolic flows have been shown to correlate strongly with fetal distress and intrauterine death.

See Chapter 6, *Obstetrics by Ten Teachers,* 19th edition.

5 Prenatal diagnosis

a) This is an autosomal recessive disorder. Therefore if both parents are carriers, the chances of having an affected child are 1:4 in each pregnancy.
b) The most common mutation is the delta 508 mutation and this is present in 68 per cent of cases.
c) This could be diagnosed prenatally from a chorionic villus biopsy. It can also be made from an amniocentesis sample.
d) The chorionic villus biopsy can be performed any time after 10 weeks' gestation. Amniocentesis can be performed after 14 weeks' gestation.

See Chapter 7, *Obstetrics by Ten Teachers*, 19th edition.

6 Second trimester miscarriage

a) The combination of two previous losses that presented with backache would suggest mid-trimester loss.
b) A general examination should be performed to check that the woman is well. This should include the patient's vital signs: pulse, temperature and blood pressure. A temperature may suggest infection, as would a tachycardia. Abdominal examination should be performed to palpate for contractions. Fetal heart auscultation should be performed to confirm fetal viability. Initially a sterile speculum examination should be performed and a vaginal swab taken. Visualization of the cervix will determine whether it is dilating. A cervico-vaginal swab should be obtained to exclude infection. A urine sample should be obtained to exclude urinary tract infection which may precipitate uterine activity. A full blood count should be taken to look for signs of infection. An ultrasound scan should be performed to confirm viability and gestation.
c) Adequate analgesia is essential so that the patient suffers as little distress as possible. Vaginal delivery will almost always occur due to the small size of the fetus. Some of these babies will show signs of life and the parents need to be warned of this to avoid unnecessary distress. The parents should be offered contact details of support groups.

See Chapter 11, *Obstetrics by Ten Teachers*, 19th edition.

7 Antenatal obstetric complications

There are three available management options that need to be discussed with the patient. These are:

a) Elective Caesarean section.
b) External cephalic version (ECV).
c) Vaginal breech delivery.

The candidate would be expected to take a brief obstetric history. This would be to determine whether there were any factors in the history that would be a contraindication to vaginal breech delivery or ECV.

The Term Breech Trial demonstrated that there was a reduction in the perinatal mortality and morbidity with elective Caesarean section over vaginal breech delivery. However, there are some factors that would increase the strength of recommendation for a Caesarean section, these being a large or small baby, a small pelvis on pelvimetry, previous Caesarean section and extended fetal neck.

External cephalic version is carried out at 36–37 weeks' gestation. The procedure has been shown to reduce the number of Caesarean sections due to breech presentation. Contraindications to ECV are placenta praevia, oilgohydramnios, previous Caesarean section, multiple gestation and pre-eclampsia. The risks of the procedure, which need to be outlined, are placental abruption, premature rupture of the fetal membranes, cord accident, transplacental haemorrhage and fetal bradycardia.

Vaginal breech delivery is still an acceptable option if the mother understands the increased risks to the fetus. There are a number of factors that increase the likelihood of a successful breech delivery: normal-size baby, flexed neck, multiparous, breech deeply engaged, and positive mental attitude of the woman.

See Chapter 8, *Obstetrics by Ten Teachers*, 19th edition.

8 Twins and higher-order multiple gestations

a) Monozygotic twins arise from a single fertilized ovum that splits into two identical structures. The type of monozygotic twins depends on how long after conception this splitting occurs.
b) Chorionicity refers to the number of placentae shared among a given set of twins. The most reliable time to determine chorionicity is at the end of the first trimester. In dichorionic twins there is extension of the placental tissue into the base of the intertwin membrane. This is known as the 'lambda' sign. In monochorionic twins this sign is absent and the membrane joins the uterine wall in a t-shape.
c) There is an increased risk of intrauterine growth restriction compared with singleton pregnancies. The risk of fetal anomaly is greater in all twin pregnancies; however, the risk is highest in monochorionic twin pregnancies. There is an increased risk of preterm labour in all twin pregnancies. The overall perinatal mortality rate for twins is six times higher than for singleton pregnancies.
d) Monochorionic twins carry a risk of twin-to-twin transfusion syndrome. This occurs due to vascular anastomoses between the two fetoplacental circulations. This is a potential dangerous complication that without treatment will lead to miscarriage or severe preterm delivery in 90 per cent of cases.

See Chapter 9, *Obstetrics by Ten Teachers*, 19th edition.

9 Disorders of placentation

a) The most likely diagnosis based on the blood picture is pre-eclampsia.
b) Any three of the following:

   1 Blood pressure >140/90.
   2 Hypereflexia.
   3 Clonus.
   4 Papilloedema.
   5 Visual disturbances.
   6 Small for gestational age.

c) Any of the following three:

   1 Eclampsia.
   2 Cerebrovascular accidents.
   3 Renal failure.
   4 Adult respiratory distress syndrome.

d) Treat blood pressure with antihypertensives. Administer steroids to accelerate lung maturity. Monitor fetus and indices and consider delivery with worsening indices. Inform the neonatal unit about impeding delivery.
e) She should have an ultrasound scan for fetal growth and liquor volume. Umbilical artery Dopplers should be performed.

See Chapter 10, *Obstetrics by Ten Teachers*, 19th edition.

10 Preterm labour

a) The first investigation that should be initiated is genital tract swabs. This may guide antibiotic therapy if required. An ultrasound can give valuable information on the amniotic fluid volume. There is a direct correlation between the amount of amniotic fluid and the time to labour. Maternal well-being should be regularly assessed; this should include pulse and blood pressure and some advocate serial C-reactive protein and white cell count. Fetal well-being should also be regularly monitored with cardiotocography.

b) Neonatal survival can rarely occur at 23 weeks, is possible at 24–25 weeks and likely after 26 weeks.

c) Any women delivering after preterm rupture of the fetal membranes is at increased risk of endometritis and postpartum haemorrhage. Therefore prophylactic antibiotics should be considered.

d) This woman should be advised that there are non-modifiable and modifiable risk factors, and that she is at 20 per cent risk of preterm birth in view of her history. Smoking is an independent risk factor and cessation of smoking will reduce her risk. Drug abuse is also linked to preterm labour and can be stopped. An inter-pregnancy interval of less than 1 year is associated with an increased risk and therefore delaying subsequent pregnancies may reduce the risk. An early dating scan should be arranged to ensure precise assessment of fetal gestational age. Vaginal swabs should be taken and tested for bacterial vaginosis (BV) and Group B streptococcus. Treatment of women with BV in high-risk populations has been shown to reduce the preterm birth rate by 60 per cent.

See Chapter 11, *Obstetrics by Ten Teachers*, 19th edition.

11 Medical diseases of pregnancy

a) The most common acquired cardiac lesion is mitral stenosis.

b) Prematurity is a common effect of cardiac disease. This can be either iatrogenic or because the fetus is small for gestational age. There is also an increase in maternal mortality; however, this varies dependent on the cardiac lesion. There is also a 5 per cent risk that the fetus will have a congenital heart defect.

c) Induction of labour should be avoided unless for obstetric indications. Prophylactic antibiotics should be given to prevent bacterial endocarditis. A close monitoring of fluid balance should be initiated. Anaesthesia should be discussed with a senior anaesthetist. The second stage of labour should be kept short.

See Chapter 12, *Obstetrics by Ten Teachers*, 19th edition.

12 Perinatal infections

a) HIV is a single-stranded retrovirus that binds to CD4 receptors.

b) T-helper lymphocyctes, macrophages, dendritic cells and microglia cells present CD4 receptors.

c) There are two main strategies used in the treatment of HIV. If there is no evidence of immunodeficiency then antiretroviral drug therapy is commenced as highly active retroviral therapy. This is a combination of several drugs that include nucleoside reverse transcriptase inhibitors, a non-nucleoside reverse transcriptase inhibitor and a protease inhibitor. If there is evidence of immunodeficiency, treatment is aimed at prevention of opportunistic infection.

d) Vertical transmission occurs in 25–40 per cent of pregnancies if there are no interventions to reduce the risk. The three interventions that have been shown to reduce the vertical transmission of HIV are avoiding breastfeeding, elective Caesarean section and the use of antiviral drugs in the later half of pregnancy and the neonatal period.

See Chapter 13, *Obstetrics by Ten Teachers*, 19th edition.

13 Labour

a) The chart is a partogram of X.
b) This is a partogram. It is a pictorial presentation of the process of labour.
c) The first stage of labour is defined as the time from the diagnosis of labour to full dilatation of the cervix. The second stage of labour is defined as the time from full dilatation of the cervix to the delivery of the fetus or fetuses. The third stage of labour is defined as the time from the delivery of the fetus to delivery of the placenta.
d) The diagram illustrates secondary arrest of labour due to irregular uterine contractions.
e) From the partogram the membranes are still intact as there is no liquor draining. Therefore an artificial rupture of the membranes should be performed. The patient should be examined 2 hours after this. If there is still no progress, syntocinon should be commenced.

See Chapter 14, *Obstetrics by Ten Teachers*, 19th edition.

14 Operative interventions in obstetrics

a) The instrument is a ventouse.
b) It is used for delay in the second stage, fetal distress in the second stage and maternal conditions requiring a short second stage.
c) It is contraindicated in face presentation, gestation less than 34 weeks and marked active bleeding from the fetal blood sample site.
d) Maternal complications include vaginal lacerations and cervical injury.
e) Possible fetal complications include chignon, cephalohaematoma, neonatal jaundice and lacerations of the fetal scalp.

See Chapter 15, *Obstetrics by Ten Teachers*, 19th edition.

15 Obstetric emergencies

a) Postpartum haemorrhage is defined as excess blood loss (1000 mL) in the first 24 hours after delivery.
b) You would:
   • Call for help.
   • Massage the uterus.
   • Gain intravenous access.
   • Give high-dose syntocinon.
   • Determine the cause of the bleeding and deal with it.

c) The four most common causes of postpartum haemorrhage can be remembered with the simple:
   Tone – uterine atony.
   Trauma – check for injury to vagina, perineum and uterine tears.
   Tissue – check placenta completely removed.
   Thrombin – clotting disorders.

See Chapter 16, *Obstetrics by Ten Teachers*, 19th edition.

16 The puerperium

a) The mostly likely diagnosis in a woman presenting with this history is a pulmonary embolism.
b) The patient may complain of a cough and haemoptysis. She may also complain of a swollen, painful calf secondary to a deep vein thrombosis (DVT) of the leg. There may be a family history of DVT or PE.

c) Examination may reveal tachypnoea, raised jugular venous pressure and right ventricular heave. The patient's calf may also be swollen and painful, suggesting a DVT.

d) A chest x-ray should be performed. This is usually normal; however, it excludes other causes of breathlessness. An electrocardiogram (ECG) should be performed, but this may also be normal except for a sinus tachycardia. Arterial blood gases would show hypoxaemia and hypercapnia. The definitive test for a pulmonary embolism (PE) is a V/Q scan. This will demonstrate a ventilation/perfusion mismatch.

e) The initial treatment is with intravenous heparin or subcuticular low molecular-weight heparin.

See Chapter 17, *Obstetrics by Ten Teachers*, 19th edition.

17 Psychiatric disorders in pregnancy and the puerperium

a) The mostly likely diagnosis is postpartum depression.

b) She may complain of early morning waking, a loss of appetite, low energy, lack of enjoyment, anxiety, thoughts of self-harm.

c) There are three main treatment options. These include remedy of social factors. However, several randomized trials have demonstrated the benefits of non-directive counselling from specially trained midwives and health visitors. If pharmacotherapy is deemed necessary, tricyclic antidepressants or SSRI are widely used. There is evidence to support their safety in post-natal breastfeeding women.

d) A psychiatric disorder specific to pregnancy is puerperal psychosis.

e) Treatment is aimed at dealing with the acute psychotic event. This can be achieved with the use of neuroleptics such a haloperidol or chlorpromazine. If there is a significant manic component to the presentation, lithium carbonate should be initiated. Electroconvulsive therapy is an option in women with severe depressive psychosis. Antidepressants are used as a second-line therapy.

See Chapter 18, *Obstetrics by Ten Teachers*, 19th edition.

18 Neonatology

a) There are many circumstances where a trained resuscitator should be present, including:
Preterm deliveries.
Vaginal breech delivery.
Significant fetal distress.
Serious fetal abnormality.
Rotational forceps.
Caesarean section.

b) The Apgar score is a tool that was developed to assist the recognition of an infant who is failing to make a successful transition to extrauterine life. It has five separate categories that are scored 0, 1 or 2 depending on the observation of the neonate, to give a maximum score of 10. The categories are appearance (central trunk colour), pulse rate, response to stimulus, muscle tone and respiratory effort. The scores should be recorded at 1 minute and 5 minutes unless there is a problem, in which case further observation should be recorded.

c) The baby should be dried, wrapped in a warm, dry towel and placed under a radiant heat source. The process of drying often provides enough stimulus to induce breathing. If there is no response, commence active resuscitation using five inflation breaths via a bag and mask and summon help.

d) Level 2 intensive care is provided by specially trained nursing staff who care for two babies at one time. Examples would include babies requiring parenteral nutrition, having apnoeic attacks or requiring oxygen treatment and weighing less than 1500 g.

See Chapter 19, *Obstetrics by Ten Teachers*, 19th edition.

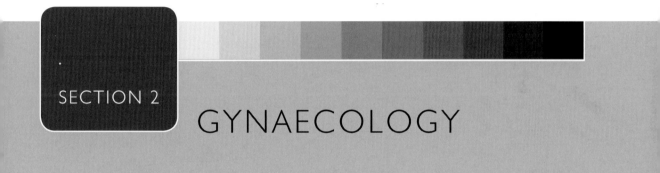

GYNAECOLOGY

EXTENDED MATCHING QUESTIONS

QUESTIONS

1 Embryology

A Mesonephric ducts

B Paramesonephric duct

C Müllerian system

D Sinovaginal bulbs

E Genital tubercle

F Genital folds

G Urethral folds of the cloaca

H Genital ridge

For each description below, choose the SINGLE most appropriate answer from the above list of options. Each option may be used once, more than once, or not at all.

1 Develop(s) into the uterus, cervix and proximal 2/3 of the vagina.

2 Form(s) the ovary.

3 Develop(s) into the distal one third of the vagina.

4 Develop(s) into the labia minora.

2 Anatomy and physiology

A Aorta

B Internal iliac vein

C Renal vein

D Vena cava

E Superficial inguinal and femoral nodes

F Obturator, internal and external iliac nodes

G Para-aortic nodes

H External iliac vein

For each description below, choose the SINGLE most appropriate answer from the above list of options. Each option may be used once, more than once, or not at all.

1 Lymphatic drainage of the ovary.

2 Lymphatic drainage of the lower vagina and vulva.

3 Lymphatic drainage of the upper vagina and cervix.

4 Venous drainage from the left ovarian vein.

3 Normal and abnormal sexual development and puberty

A Cloacal cells
B 17-Hydroxyprogesterone
C Wolffian duct
D Testosterone
E Dihydrotestosterone
F Leydig cells
G SRY region
H Sertoli cells

For each description below, choose the SINGLE most appropriate answer from the above list of options. Each option may be used once, more than once, or not at all.

1 Responsible for the production of testicular development factor (TDF).
2 Responsible for the production of Müllerian inhibitor.
3 Responsible for the production of testosterone.
4 Hormone responsible for the development of the vas deferens, epididymis and seminal vesicles.

4 Disorders of the menstrual cycle

A Adenomyosis
B Stress incontinence
C Endometrial polyp
D Malignancy of the cervix
E Fibroids
F Pelvic inflammatory disease
G Endometrial malignancy
H Uterine prolapse

For each description below, choose the SINGLE most appropriate answer from the above list of options. Each option may be used once, more than once, or not at all.

1 Intermenstrual bleeding.
2 Post-coital bleeding.
3 Post-menopausal bleeding.
4 Painful periods.

5 Disorders of the menstrual cycle

A Transcervical resection of the endometrium
B Vaginal hysterectomy
C Endometrial ablation
D Hysteroscopy and curettage
E Manchester repair
F Myomectomy
G Abdominal hysterectomy
H Mirena

For each description below, choose the SINGLE most appropriate answer from the above list of options. Each option may be used once, more than once, or not at all.

1 A procedure for the investigation of menorrhagia but not a treatment.
2 An outpatient procedure that destroys the endometrium and fibroids up to 4 cm in diameter.
3 A procedure for women with fibroids who want to retain their fertility.
4 A definitive treatment for menorrhagia refractive to other treatments, if the uterus is not enlarged and ovarian conservation is required.

6 Disorders of the menstrual cycle

A Cyclical norethisterone
B Combined oral contraceptive pill
C LNG-IUS
D Mefenamic acid
E Tranexamic acid
F Gonadotrophin-releasing hormone analogues
G Danazol
H Gestrinone

For each description below, choose the SINGLE most appropriate answer from the above list of options. Each option may be used once, more than once, or not at all.

1 The five-year prolonged exposure of the endometrium to progesterone to cause thinning of the endometrium and lighter menses.
2 This reduces production of prostaglandin E2 and reduces loss by up to 25 per cent.
3 This is to be taken from days 5 to 26 in anovulatory dysfunctional uterine bleeding; it regulates the cycle and promotes secretory endometrium in the second half of the cycle.
4 This promotes coagulation and reduces menstrual loss by 40 per cent.

7 Infertility

A Clomid
B Anovulation
C Oligospermia
D Azoospermia
E Polycystic ovary syndrome
F Chlamydia
G Androgen-secreting tumour
H Puregon

For each description below, choose the SINGLE most appropriate answer from the above list of options. Each option may be used once, more than once, or not at all.

1 This is associated with a raised free androgen index, low sex hormone-binding globulin and raised testosterone.
2 The most common cause of tubal disease in the Western world.
3 The only treatment is donor insemination.
4 An oral treatment for anovulation.

8 Disorders of early pregnancy

A Threatened miscarriage
B Silent miscarriage
C Incomplete miscarriage
D Ectopic pregnancy
E Hydatidiform mole
F Heterotropic pregnancy
G Choriocarcinoma
H Septic miscarriage

For each description below, choose the SINGLE most appropriate answer from the above list of options. Each option may be used once, more than once, or not at all.

1 The abnormal proliferation of trophoblastic tissue with or without embryonic tissue.
2 The partial expulsion of products of conception with products of conception seen measuring 65 mm in diameter on ultrasound scan.
3 Bleeding in pregnancy, <24 weeks' gestation with fetal heart visible on ultrasound scan and closed cervical os.
4 Light bleeding, pelvic pain, shoulder-tip pain, 7 weeks' gestation, empty uterus on ultrasound and fluid in pouch of Douglas.

9 Benign diseases of the cervix

A Squamous metaplasia
B Columnar epithelium
C Moderate dyskaryosis
D Severe dyskaryosis
E Borderline nuclear change
F Mild dyskaryosis
G Glandular atypia
H Arias–Stella change

For each description below, choose the SINGLE most appropriate answer from the above list of options. Each option may be used once, more than once, or not at all.

1 CIN1.
2 CIN2.
3 CIN3.
4 CGIN.

10 Benign diseases of the uterus

A Leiomyosarcoma
B Pedunculated leiomyoma
C Hyaline degeneration
D Adenomyosis
E Red degeneration
F Endometriosis
G Brenner's tumour
H Calcified degeneration

For each description below, choose the SINGLE most appropriate answer from the above list of options. Each option may be used once, more than once, or not at all.

1 This occurs as a result of disruption of blood supply (typically pregnancy related).
2 Necrosis and cystic formation due to outgrowth of blood supply.
3 Fibroid change that is usually a post-menopausal manifestation.
4 Malignant change that accounts for >1 per cent of fibroids.

11 Endometriosis and adenomyosis

A Transcervical resection of the endometrium
B Laser ablation to endometrial deposits
C Hydrothermal ablation
D Total abdominal hysterectomy and bilateral salpingo-oophorectomy
E Combined oral contraceptive pill
F Vaginal hysterectomy
G Conservative management
H Surgical drainage and post-operative gonadotrophin-releasing hormone (GnRH) antagonist treatment

For each description below, choose the SINGLE most appropriate answer from the above list of options. Each option may be used once, more than once, or not at all.

1 Treatment for minimal endometriosis to improve chances of conception in patient with infertility.
2 Definitive treatment for Stage IV endometriosis, obliterated rectovaginal septum and bilateral endometriomas.
3 Asymptomatic endometriosis found on routine laparoscopy for sterilization.
4 Symptomatic endometriosis in a twenty three-year-old woman who wants children but is currently not contemplating pregnancy.

12 Benign diseases of the ovary

A Fibroma
B Serous cystadenoma
C Teratoma
D Endometroid tumour
E Clear cell tumour
F Granulosa cell tumour
G Brenner's tumour
H Mucinous cystadenoma

For each description below, choose the SINGLE most appropriate answer from the above list of options. Each option may be used once, more than once, or not at all.

1 A unilocular cyst with papillous processes usually occurring unilaterally.
2 A large unilateral multiloculated cyst lined by columnar epithelium and complicated with pseudomyxoma peritonii.
3 A large cyst usually containing unclotted blood with a ground-glass appearance on ultrasound.
4 This has a solid appearance with islands of transitional epithelium in dense fibrotic stroma.

13 Malignant disease of the uterus and cervix

A Subtotal abdominal hysterectomy
B Cold coagulation
C Wertheim's hysterectomy
D LLETZ (large loop excision of the transformation zone)
E Pelvic exenteration
F Bilateral salpingo-oophorectomy
G Palliative treatment
H Wertheim's hysterectomy and radiotherapy

For each description below, choose the SINGLE most appropriate answer from the above list of options. Each option may be used once, more than once, or not at all.

1 CIN2.
2 Ectopy.
3 Stage 1B cervical cancer.
4 Stage 2 cervical cancer.

14 Carcinoma of the ovary and Fallopian tube

A Laser laparoscopy
B Vaginal hysterectomy
C Total abdominal hysterectomy (TAH), bilateral salpingo-oophorectomy (BSO) and omentectomy
D Subtotal hysterectomy carboplatin
E Unilateral salpingo-oophorectomy and peritoneal washings
F TCRE
G Wertheim's hysterectomy
H Debulking surgery and subsequent or cisplatin/paclitaxel chemotherapy

For each description below, choose the SINGLE most appropriate answer from the above list of options. Each option may be used once, more than once, or not at all.

1 Stage 1B ovarian cancer.
2 Stage 3 epithelioid tumour.
3 Unilateral borderline tumour.
4 Endometriosis.

15 Infections in gynaecology

A Candida
B Chlamydia
C Bacterial vaginosis
D Trichomoniasis
E Herpes
F Syphilis
G Human immunodeficiency virus (HIV)
H Gonorrhoea

For each description below, choose the SINGLE most appropriate answer from the above list of options. Each option may be used once, more than once, or not at all.

1 A sexually transmitted disease typified by genital ulcers and painful vesicles.
2 A non-sexually transmitted infection typified by itchy, sore vagina with a white 'curdy' discharge.
3 A non-sexually transmitted disease typified by an offensive fishy discharge.
4 A sexually transmitted disease typified by Gram-negative diplococci, and colonizing columnar and cuboidal epithelium; 50 per cent are found asymptomatically.

16 Urogynaecology

A Urodynamic stress incontinence   **D** Bladder diverticulum   **G** Detrusor overactivity
B Normal bladder function   **E** Sensory urgency   **H** Detrusor–sphincter dyssynergia
C Poor detrusor contraction   **F** Bladder outflow obstruction

For each description below, choose the SINGLE most appropriate answer from the above list of options. Each option may be used once, more than once, or not at all.

1   Detrusor pressure rise of >15 cm of water during filling associated with urgency.
2   A voiding detrusor pressure of 10 cm of water and flow rate of 5 mL per second.
3   Leakage on coughing in the absence of detrusor contraction.
4   Voiding detrusor pressure of >70 cm of water and peak flow rate of 5 mL second.

17 Uterovaginal prolapse

A Anterior repair   **D** Posterior repair   **G** Ring pessary
B Shelf pessary   **E** Vaginal hysterectomy   **H** Manchester repair
C Sacrospinous fixation   **F** Sacrocolpopexy

For each description below, choose the SINGLE most appropriate answer from the above list of options. Each option may be used once, more than once, or not at all.

1   The treatment for vault prolapse in a frail elderly woman who would not be suitable for surgery.
2   Amputation of the cervical stump and plication of the uterosacral and cardinal ligaments.
3   The treatment of choice for a symptomatic cystocele with no history of incontinence in a fifty-year-old, sexually active woman.
4   Treatment of vault prolapse in an elderly woman with multiple previous abdominal surgery who is not sexually active.

18 The menopause

A Tibolone   **D** Norplant   **G** Vagifem
B Medroxyprogesterone acetate   **E** Conjugated equine oestrogen   **H** Implanon
C Transdermal patch containing 50 mg of oestrogen   **F** Echinacea

For each description below, choose the SINGLE most appropriate answer from the above list of options. Each option may be used once, more than once, or not at all.

1   An oral hormone replacement therapy (HRT) preparation that is converted to oestrone by hepatic enzymes resulting in a plasma oestradiol (E2)/oestrone ratio of 1:2.
2   A lipid-soluble preparation maintaining an E2/oestrone ratio of 2:1, which is similar to pre-menopausal physiological status.
3   An HRT with mild androgenic side effects, which may have a beneficial effect on low libido.
4   An essential part of HRT to reduce the risk of endometrial hyperplasia in women with a uterus.

19 Common gynaecological procedures and medicolegal aspects of gynaecology

Surgical complications:

A TCRE
B Tension-free vaginal tape (TVT)
C Marsupialization of Bartholin's abscess

D Posterior repair
E Cystoscopy
F Laparoscopy

G Abdominal hysterectomy for extensive endometriosis
H Flexible hysteroscopy

For each description below, choose the SINGLE most appropriate answer from the above list of options. Each option may be used once, more than once, or not at all.

1 Gas embolism.
2 Ureteric injury.
3 Damage to the bladder.
4 Uterine perforation.

EMQ ANSWERS

1 Embryology

1 B   2 H   3 D   4 G

The paramesonephric (Müllerian) ducts develop into the uterus, cervix and upper 2/3 of the vagina, while in the female the mesonephric (Wolffian) ducts regress. The sinovaginal bulbs develop as outgrowths that canalize and form the distal portion of the vagina below the level of the hymen. The ovary is derived from three components: the genital ridge, the underlying mesoderm and the primitive germ cells. The genital tubercle forms the clitoris. The cloacal folds anteriorly are called the urethral folds which form the labia minora, and the labioscrotal folds of the cloacal membrane form the labia majora.

See Chapter 2, *Gynaecology by Ten Teachers*, 19th edition.

2 Anatomy and physiology

1 G   2 E   3 F   4 C

Lymphatic drainage of the ovary is via a plexus of vessels lying in the infundibulopelvic folds to the para-aortic node on both sides of the midline. The lymphatic drainage of the lower third of the vagina follows that of the vulva to the superficial inguinal and femoral nodes, while the upper portion of the vagina follows that of the cervix to the obturator, internal and external iliac nodes. The venous drainage of the ovary is to the renal vein on the left and inferior vena cava on the right.

See Chapter 2, *Gynaecology by Ten Teachers*, 19th edition.

3 Normal and abnormal sexual development and puberty

1 G   2 H   3 F   4 D

The *SRY* gene lies on the short arm of the Y chromosome and is responsible for determination of testicular development as it produces TDF. TDF stimulates the Sertoli cells of the undifferentiated gonad to produce Müllerian inhibitor. The Leydig cells produce testosterone, which promotes development of the Wolffian ducts into the vas deferens, epididymis and seminal vesicles.

See Chapter 3, *Gynaecology by Ten Teachers*, 19th edition.

4 Disorders of the menstrual cycle

1 C   2 D   3 G   4 A

Abnormal bleeding outside the normal menstrual cycle should always be investigated. Intermenstrual bleeding is commonly associated with an endometrial polyp or luteal phase insufficiency. Post-coital bleeding should always be investigated by visualization of the cervix to exclude a cervical malignancy. Post-menopausal bleeding should be considered to be endometrial carcinoma until this has been excluded by either ultrasound and endometrial sampling or hysteroscopy and curettage. Adenomyosis causes painful periods and is typified by a tender, bulky uterus.

See Chapter 5, *Gynaecology by Ten Teachers*, 19th edition.

5 Disorders of the menstrual cycle

1 D   **2** C   **3** F   **4** B

Hysteroscopy and endometrial curettage is useful to gain a view of the uterine cavity and histology of the endometrium. The endometrium can be either resected (transcervical resection of the endometrium (TCRE)) or ablated using microwaves, hot water or a balloon filled with heated solutions. Any of these methods can result in reduced menstrual loss or amenorrhoea to various degrees. Myomectomy can be performed to remove large fibroids to allow symptomatic relief without removal of the uterus, thus retaining a woman's fertility. Pregnancy is contraindicated after TCRE or ablation. Hysterectomy is the definitive treatment for menorrhagia. The route is determined by the size of the uterus, the degree of uterine descent and the necessity for oopherectomy.

See Chapter 5, *Gynaecology by Ten Teachers*, 19th edition.

6 Disorders of the menstrual cycle

1 C   **2** D   **3** A   **4** E

The levonorgestrel intrauterine system (LNG-IUS) is an intrauterine device with a sleeve impregnated with slow-release levonorgestrel (progesterone). Prolonged exposure of the endometrium to progesterone causes thinning/decidualization of the endometrium and reduces menstrual loss. Cyclical administration of progesterone, such as norethisterone, causes the endometrium to remain secretory until withdrawal of the progesterone, which results in menstruation. Antiprostaglandins, such as mefenamic acid, are non-steroidal anti-inflammatory drug derivatives and inhibit prostaglandin formation, whereas antifibrinolytics, such as tranexamic acid, inhibit lysis of formed clots. Both are useful in reducing loss in the regular cycle.

See Chapter 5, *Gynaecology by Ten Teachers*, 19th edition.

7 Infertility

1 E   **2** F   **3** D   **4** A

Polycystic ovary syndrome is a condition associated with insulin resistance. Women are typically but not always overweight, hirsute and have acne. The hormone profile of these women typically shows elevated androgens and a low sex hormone-binding globulin. Chlamydial infection is the most common cause of pelvic inflammatory disease and tubal factor infertility in the West. Men suffering from azoospermia have no sperm to be harvested and hence can have children only either by adoption or donor insemination. Anovulation can be treated orally with Clomid or by intramuscular gonadotrophins (e.g. Puregon).

See Chapter 8, *Gynaecology by Ten Teachers*, 19th edition.

8 Disorders of early pregnancy

1 E   **2** C   **3** A   **4** D

Molar pregnancies can be either partial or complete depending on whether embryonic tissue also develops. Incomplete miscarriage is associated with retained products of conception on ultrasound, whereas the uterus is empty after a complete miscarriage. If a viable pregnancy is confirmed on ultrasound after bleeding, it is defined as a threatened miscarriage. Ectopic pregnancies are typified by unilateral pain, blood in the pelvis, which causes diaphragmatic irritation, and pain referred to the shoulder tip.

See Chapter 9, *Gynaecology by Ten Teachers*, 19th edition.

9 Benign diseases of the cervix

1 F   **2** C   **3** D   **4** G

Dyskaryosis is a cytological diagnosis made on a cervical smear. Cervical intraepithelial neoplasia (CIN) is a histological diagnosis made on biopsy of cervical tissue. Mild dyskaryosis is analogous to CIN1, moderate dyskaryosis to CIN2 and severe dyskaryosis to CIN3. Glandular atypia occurs in the columnar cells of the endocervical canal and is associated with cervical glandular intraepithelial neoplasia (CGIN) and adenocarcinoma.
See Chapter 10, *Gynaecology by Ten Teachers*, 19th edition.

10 Benign diseases of the uterus

1 E   **2** C   **3** H   **4** A

Fibroids can undergo various forms of change. A sudden loss of blood supply causes pain and red degeneration typically seen in pregnancy. Hyaline degeneration occurs when a fibroid slowly outgrows its blood supply, resulting in necrosis and cyst formation. After the menopause, fibroids may calcify. Rarely, leiomyosarcoma can develop from fibroids.
See Chapter 10, *Gynaecology by Ten Teachers*, 19th edition.

11 Endometriosis and adenomyosis

1 B   **2** D   **3** G   **4** E

Endometriosis is a benign condition that has various treatments depending on the clinical situation. Asymptomatic endometriosis requires no treatment at all. The exogenous endometrial tissue is susceptible to endogenous oestrogen and the menstrual cycle. Mild to moderate endometriosis can be treated by administration of exogenous hormones, such as the combined oral contraceptive pill or GnRH agonists to downregulate the hypothalamic– pituitary–ovarian axis. Laser ablation to mild endometriosis has been shown to improve symptoms and the chances of conception in women with sub-fertility. Once a woman's family is complete and there is extensive symptomatic disease, definitive treatment is necessary along with bilateral oophorectomy.
See Chapter 11, *Gynaecology by Ten Teachers*, 19th edition.

12 Benign diseases of the ovary

1 B   **2** H   **3** D   **4** G

Ultrasound can be helpful in differentiating benign tumours. USS characterizes the morphology of the cyst, presence of bilateral tumours, ascites and omental deposits. In conjunction with a CA125 and age, a relative malignancy index (RMI) can be calculated. Certain cysts have a characteristic appearance. Serous cystadenomas are usually unilocular with papillary processes. Mucinous cystadenoma has a multiloculated appearance. Endometriomas are filled with altered blood, giving a typical ground-glass appearance on ultrasound, whereas fibromas are solid tumours that on ultrasound look similar in appearance to fibroids. More often, histological classification is necessary to determine the origin and nature of the tumour.
See Chapter 12, *Gynaecology by Ten Teachers*, 19th edition.

13 Malignant disease of the uterus and cervix

1 D   **2** B   **3** C   **4** H

Cervical ectopy is not a pre-malignant condition. It can be left alone if it is asymptomatic in the presence of a normal smear and colposcopy. If it is symptomatic, then coagulation can be used. Pre-clinical disease that invades to a depth of <3 mm and width of 7 mm can be safely treated with local excision (LLETZ). Treatment of clinical disease is usually with surgery, radiotherapy or both. If the disease is confined to the cervix, surgery or radiotherapy can be used. Once it has spread outside the cervix, radiotherapy is the main treatment modality.
See Chapter 14, *Gynaecology by Ten Teachers*, 19th edition.

14 Carcinoma of the ovary and Fallopian tube

1 C   **2** H   **3** E   **4** A

Stage 1b is confined to both ovaries with no ascites or tumour on the external surface of the ovary and an intact capsule. In this case, TAH and BSO and omentectomy are sufficient. After Stage 1B, chemotherapy is also required. Unilateral borderline tumours can be treated by removing the affected ovary and taking peritoneal washings to check for spread. However, if the patient's family is complete and there is a suspicion of malignancy, TAH and BSO and omental biopsy may be more prudent. Endometriosis is a benign condition and can be ablated with a laser or diathermy.
See Chapter 12, *Gynaecology by Ten Teachers*, 19th edition.

15 Infections in gynaecology

1 E   **2** A   **3** C   **4** H

Primary genital herpes is a sexually transmitted condition that presents with painful ulcers and vesicles, often with urinary retention due to pain. Candida is not sexually transmitted and is a common condition presenting with a white discharge and red, sore vagina, compared with bacterial vaginosis, which has a typical 'fishy' odour and frothy discharge. Gonorrhoea and chlamydia are often asymptomatic. Chlamydia is the most common cause of pelvic inflammatory disease (PID) in the West, but is diagnosed by enzyme-linked immunosorbent assay (ELISA), whereas gonorrhoea can be diagnosed on microscopy.
See Chapter 15, *Gynaecology by Ten Teachers*, 19th edition.

16 Urogynaecology

1 G   **2** C   **3** A   **4** F

A rise in detrusor pressure associated with urgency is diagnostic of detrusor overactivity. Urodynamic stress incontinence is diagnosed in the absence of a detrusor contraction. A flow rate of 5 mL per second is reduced. In the presence of a high detrusor pressure, this would indicate a bladder outflow obstruction. If the detrusor pressure was low and the flow rate also low, poor detrusor function would be more likely.
See Chapter 16, *Gynaecology by Ten Teachers*, 19th edition.

17 Uterovaginal prolapse

1 B   **2** H   **3** A   **4** C

Surgery is unsuitable in frail women who could not tolerate general or regional anaesthesia, so a pessary would be more appropriate. The Manchester repair is an operation that used to be performed for prolapse with an elongated cervix. It involved cervical amputation, anterior and posterior repair, and shortening the cardinal ligaments. Anterior repair is an effective treatment for cystocele but is not effective in treating stress incontinence. Abdominal surgery for vault prolapse (sacrocolpopexy) should be avoided if the patient is frail or has multiple previous abdominal procedures (concerns about adhesions). Sacrospinous fixation is a vaginal procedure for vault prolapse and has less morbidity associated.

See Chapter 17, *Gynaecology by Ten Teachers*, 19th edition.

18 The menopause

1 E   **2** C   **3** A   **4** B

Hormone replacement therapy can be oestrogen alone in hysterectomized women, or oestrogen and progesterone in women with a uterus. Oestrogen can be taken orally and pass through the first-pass metabolism, or through transdermal patches, which will avoid hepatic enzymes. Tibolone has mild androgenic side effects and is useful in women with a low libido. Progesterone in various forms (e.g. medroxyprogesterone acetate) is necessary in women with a uterus to prevent endometrial hyperplasia.

See Chapter 18, *Gynaecology by Ten Teachers*, 19th edition.

19 Common gynaecological procedures and medicolegal aspects of gynaecology

1 F   **2** G   **3** B   **4** A

Gas embolism can occur after laparoscopy, although it is rare. Women are usually informed of the risk of injury to the bowel or aorta from Veress needle insertion during the consent process, trochar insertion and operative laparoscopy. Endometriosis can cause tethering of the ureter to the parametrium, thus increasing the risk of ureteric injury at hysterectomy. Bladder perforation is said to occur in 1–5 per cent of TVTs. Cystoscopy is routinely performed and, if recognized, the trochars can be removed and reinserted correctly and a draining catheter left for several days. Uterine perforation and even hysterectomy are possible at TCRE. This is reduced if rollerball or endometrial ablation is performed instead.

See Chapter 19, *Gynaecology by Ten Teachers*, 19th edition.

CHAPTER 7

MULTIPLE CHOICE QUESTIONS

QUESTIONS

Please answer True (T) or False (F) to the following statements.

The gynaecological history and examination

1   **With regard to clinical examination of the gynaecological patient:**
a) Abdominal examination is mandatory as part of the gynaecological examination.
b) A chaperone is always needed for intimate examinations.
c) Palpation below a pelvic mass is possible.
d) Shifting dullness and fluid thrill can be seen due to urinary retention.
e) Bidigital examination can determine whether a pelvic mass is ovarian or uterine in origin.

Embryology and anatomy

2   **The following statements apply to the human female pelvis:**
a) The Fallopian tubes are lined by cilia to aid egg transport.
b) The middle portion of the Fallopian tube is called the ampulla.
c) In its upper portion the ureter lies anterior to the ovary.
d) The ovary is attached to the uterus by the round ligament.
e) The ovary has a central medulla of loose connective tissue and an outer cortex covered by cuboidal germinal epithelium.

3   **The peritoneum overlies the following structures in whole or in part:**
a) Bladder.
b) Rectum.
c) Uterus.
d) Ovary.
e) Ureter.

Normal and abnormal sexual development and puberty

4   The following have an XX karyotype:
a) Congenital adrenal hyperplasia.
b) Rokitansky's syndrome.
c) Turner's syndrome.
d) 5 alpha-reductase deficiency.
e) Androgen insensitivity.

The normal menstrual cycle

5   Within the follicular phase of the menstrual cycle:
a) The follicular phase is always 14 days long to allow development of the follicle.
b) Follicle-stimulating hormone (FSH) stimulates the granulosa cells to produce oestrogen.
c) Each cycle usually involves the development, growth and ovulation of a single follicle.
d) Follicles over 20 mm need to be drained with ultrasound guidance.
e) Oestrogen and inhibin have a positive feedback on the pituitary to release FSH and luteinizing hormone (LH).

6   In relation to ovulation:
a) LH stimulates the thecal cells of the ovary to produce oestrogen.
b) FSH induces a rise in LH receptors.
c) Ovulation occurs 4 days after the LH surge.
d) The release of an oocyte from the follicle requires a sperm to lyse the follicle membrane, and results in ovulation.
e) Ovulation can be confirmed by measurement of LH on day 14.

7   Within the luteal phase of the menstrual cycle:
a) The predominant hormone in the luteal phase is progesterone.
b) The granulosa cells of the corpus luteum have a rich vascular supply and have a yellow pigment owing to accumulation of cholesterol.
c) The luteal phase varies in duration depending on the time taken for the corpus luteum to degenerate.
d) After fertilization the corpus luteum continues to degenerate in early pregnancy.
e) Low levels of oestrogen and progesterone are the best indicators of the perimenopause.

Disorders of the menstrual cycle

8   The following are associated with menstrual disorders:
a) Endometrial polyp.
b) Endometrial simple hyperplasia.
c) Pelvic inflammatory disease.
d) Thyroid disease.
e) Diabetes.

Fertility control, contraception and absorption

9   The progesterone-only pill:
a) Has a higher failure rate in women under the age of forty than in women over the age of forty.
b) Has a lower risk of ectopic pregnancy.
c) Has a 3-hour window.
d) Has a better bleeding profile compared with the combined oral contraceptive pill (COCP).
e) Has a quicker reversibility compared with the combined oral contraceptive pill.

10 Use of the intrauterine contraceptive device (IUCD):
a) The intrauterine system (IUS) contains norethisterone.
b) The intrauterine system (Mirena) is licensed for ten years.
c) Heavy bleeding is the most common side effect with the Mirena.
d) The risk of pelvic inflammatory disease is increased with IUCD use.
e) There is an increased risk of ectopic pregnancy with IUCD use.

11 The combined oral contraceptive pill:
a) Inhibits ovulation.
b) Improves cycle control.
c) Has a 3-hour window.
d) Is relatively contraindicated in patients with acute/severe liver disease.
e) Has a risk of venous thromboembolism of 15 per 100 000 in third-generation preparations.

Subfertility

12 With regard to the investigation of the infertile couple:
a) A full hormone profile, tubal patency testing and semen analysis should be completed on all couples attending a referral for primary infertility.
b) A mid-luteal progesterone 0.25 nmol/L confirms ovulation.
c) A semen analysis should be performed prior to laparoscopy and dye to test for tubal patency.
d) Hysterosalpingogram, and laparoscopy and dye insufflation will gain similar information and either can be used to assess tubal patency in all patients.
e) A single semen analysis with a volume of 1 mL, a concentration of 10 million/mL and 30 per cent reduced motility confirms oligospermia, and serum testosterone, gonadotrophins and prolactin analysis should be performed.

Problems in early pregnancy

13 In early pregnancy:
a) Total loss of conception after fertilization is around 50–70 per cent.
b) The total rate of clinical miscarriage is around one-quarter to one-third of all pregnancies.
c) Miscarriage is much greater before 6 weeks than after 9 weeks.
d) The rate of miscarriage is the same in women over forty years of age as with women under forty.
e) The most common cause of spontaneous miscarriage is infection.

14 The following are associated with molar pregnancy:
a) Dermoid cysts.
b) Large for dates.
c) Hyperemesis.
d) Pre-eclampsia.
e) Diploidy.

15 Ectopic pregnancy:
a) Occurs in 0.5 per cent of all pregnancies.
b) Is associated with Group B streptococcus infection.
c) Is treated by laparoscopic salpingectomy if the other tube is normal.
d) Has a higher risk of persistent trophoblast if the patient has a laparoscopic salpingotomy rather than salpingectomy.
e) Cannot be managed with methotrexate if the mass is 1 cm in diameter on ultrasound.

Diseases of the ovary

16 In dermoid cysts:
a) The malignancy rate is low (around 2 per cent).
b) 50 per cent are bilateral.
c) They are often lined by embryonic mesodermal structures.
d) Struma ovarii are predominantly made of thyroid tissue.
e) Complications include torsion, chemical peritonitis and rupture.

17 In sex cord tumours:
a) All granulosa cell tumours are malignant, but are usually confined to the ovary and have a good prognosis.
b) Call–Exner bodies are pathognomonic of theca cell tumours.
c) Many theca cell tumours cause post-menopausal bleeding and endometrial carcinoma.
d) Meigs' syndrome is the combination of fibroma, ascites and pleural effusions.
e) Virilization is seen in 75 per cent of Sertoli–Leydig cell tumours.

18 The following factors on ultrasound are suspicious of malignancy:
a) A single loculated cyst of 7 cm diameter.
b) Multiple cysts around the periphery of the ovary with a dense stroma.
c) A single frond floating within a cyst.
d) Solid elements and septae.
e) Calcification and fats.

19 The following are associated with a raised alpha-fetoprotein (AFP):
a) Endodermal yolk sac tumours.
b) Granulosa cell tumours.
c) Epithelial ovarian cancer.
d) Dysgerminomas.
e) Choriocarcinoma.

Premalignant and malignant disease of the cervix

20 The following are risk factors for the development of cervical cancer:
a) Human papillomavirus (HPV) types 14, 17 and 31.
b) HPV types 16 and 18.
c) Family history of cervical cancer.
d) Smoking.
e) Previous chlamydial infection.

Malignant disease of the uterus

21 The following are risk factors for the development of endometrial cancer:
a) Obesity.
b) Diabetes.
c) Multiparity.
d) Early menopause.
e) Tamoxifen.

Diseases of the ovary

22 Regarding carcinoma of the ovary:
a) It is most common in developing countries.
b) The incidence is similar to carcinoma of the endometrium with similar prognosis.
c) The peak age is 80–90 years old.
d) The majority are epithelial in origin.
e) The mainstay of treatment is surgery and radiotherapy combined.

23 The following primary malignancies metastasize to ovary:
a) Lung.
b) Stomach.
c) Breast.
d) Thyroid.
e) Bone.

24 The following are risk factors for ovarian cancer:
a) Early menarche.
b) Early menopause.
c) Combined oral contraceptive pill usage.
d) Infertility.
e) Implanon implants.

25 The following are appropriate investigations for ovarian cancer:
a) Computed tomography (CT) of the abdomen and pelvis.
b) Barium enema.
c) Intravenous pyelogram (IVP).
d) Ultrasound scan.
e) CA 125.

26 The following are common side effects of cisplatin use:
a) Peripheral neuropathy and hearing loss.
b) Hyperkalaemia.
c) Hypomagnesaemia.
d) Renal damage.
e) Visual disturbances.

27 The following are epithelial tumours:
a) Mucinous tumour.
b) Theca cell tumour.
c) Teratoma.
d) Brenner cell tumour.
e) Androblastoma.

28 Considering dysgerminomas:
a) The peak age is over forty five years old.
b) CA 125 is elevated in 50 per cent of cases.
c) They are mainly solid rather than cystic in nature.
d) They can cause a rise in alpha-fetoprotein and hCG.
e) Immature teratomas are benign and are commonly called dermoid tumours.

Conditions affecting the vagina and vulva

29 The following are causes of pruritis vulvae:
a) Lichen sclerosus.
b) Nephrotic syndrome.
c) Atrophy.
d) Vaginal discharge.
e) Diabetes.

30 The following apply to lichen sclerosis:
a) Sites commonly affected are the labia majora and mons pubis.
b) Labial adhesions.
c) White plaques.
d) It is commonly associated with autoimmune disorders such as diabetes and pernicious anaemia.
e) Areas of dark red-brown pigmentation.

31 The following are causes of benign vulval ulcers:
a) Tertiary syphilis.
b) Chancroid.
c) Herpes.
d) HPV infection.
e) Ulcerative colitis.

32 With regard to the lower genital tract:
a) The lower genital tract is lined by stratified squamous epithelium throughout life.
b) Vaginal pH is increased under the influence of oestrogen.
c) The pH after the menopause is around 7.0.
d) Candidal infection is increased in pregnancy, with combined oral contraceptive pill usage and broad-spectrum antibiotic usage.
e) Candida is the most common cause of abnormal vaginal discharge in women of childbearing age.

33 Concerning herpes simplex virus:
a) The diagnosis is made on endocervical swabs.
b) Urinary retention and perineal pain are common presentations.
c) Reactivation of the virus occurs after colonization of neurones in Onuf's nucleus.
d) Secondary infection in pregnancy necessitates delivery by lower-segment Caesarean section.
e) Treatment with antiviral drugs is useful in established disease.

34 In relation to syphilis:
a) The causative organism is *Treponema pallidum*.
b) The TPHA is the most sensitive and specific test for syphilis.
c) Primary infection usually presents with a painful ulcer on the perineum.
d) Primary and secondary syphilis are not life threatening; however, tertiary neurosyphilis is life threatening, hence the importance of making the diagnosis.
e) Early treatment is with quadruple therapy of rifampicin, isoniazid, pyrazinamide and ethambutol.

Urogynaecology

35 The following are risk factors for the development of prolapse:
a) Nulliparity.
b) Forceps delivery.
c) Menopause.
d) Caesarean section.
e) Genetic factors.

The menopause

36 The following are absolute contraindications to taking HRT:
a) Large uterine fibroids.
b) Endometrial cancer.
c) Active liver disease.
d) Migraine with aura.
e) Otosclerosis.

37 The following are common oestrogen-related side effects to HRT:
a) Fluid retention.
b) Breast enlargement.
c) Leg cramps.
d) Dyspepsia.
e) Acne.

Psychosocial and ethical aspects of gynaecology

38 Which of the following statements are true?
a) In induced abortion, the gestation is not to exceed 26 weeks.
b) The decision can be made by any registered doctor or medical practitioner as long as they are acting in good faith.
c) Pre-operative assessment of patients before termination includes a vaginal examination to date the pregnancy and if there is any uncertainty about date, an ultrasound scan would be indicated.
d) The patient should have a chlamydia swab performed before theatre, as the incidence of chlamydia is higher in patients attending for termination of pregnancy.
e) A failed termination of pregnancy and continuation of the pregnancy is greater if termination is performed after 10 weeks.

MCQ ANSWERS

1 T, T, F, F, T

Shifting dullness and a fluid thrill are found with ascites and fluid within the peritoneal cavity.

See Chapter 1, *Gynaecology by Ten Teachers*, 19th edition.

2 T, F, F, F, T

The Fallopian tube has a lateral ampulla, middle isthmus and medial ostium. The ovary is attached to the cornua of the uterus by the ovarian ligament and to the hilum by the broad ligament. The ureter lies lateral to the ovary passing through the ovarian fossa.

See Chapter 2, *Gynaecology by Ten Teachers*, 19th edition.

3 T, T, T, F, T

The rectum is covered by the peritoneum on the front and sides in its upper third, front in its middle third and not at all in its lower third. The ovary is the only pelvic organ not covered by the peritoneum.

See Chapter 2, *Gynaecology by Ten Teachers*, 19th edition.

4 T, T, F, F, F

Turner's syndrome has XO karyotype. 5 alpha-reductase deficiency and androgen insensitivity both have XY karyotype.

See Chapter 3, *Gynaecology by Ten Teachers*, 19th edition.

5 F, T, T, F, F

The follicular phase varies in duration and this determines the cycle length (28–35 days). During each cycle, several primordial follicles develop, but only one follicle becomes dominant and continues to grow to around 20 mm in diameter. This follicle can be measured on ultrasound. It produces more oestrogen, while other follicles degenerate (undergo atresia). Ovarian cysts can grow up to 50 mm without any intervention necessary other than ultrasound observation. When cysts grow over 50 mm, there is a risk of ovarian torsion and therefore if they are persistent over 6 months' observation, drainage or cystectomy are required. Oestrogen and inhibin have a negative feedback on the production of FSH.

See Chapter 4, *Gynaecology by Ten Teachers*, 19th edition.

6 F, T, F, F, F

Luteinizing hormone stimulates the thecal cells to produce progesterone. Ovulation occurs 24 hours after the LH surge. Ovulation is caused by the enzymatic degradation of the follicle membrane by endogenous plasminogen activators and prostaglandins. Fertilization involves the degradation of the zona pellucida of the oocyte by enzymes released from the acrosome of the sperm. Ovulation can be confirmed by measuring progesterone in the mid-luteal phase.

See Chapter 4, *Gynaecology by Ten Teachers*, 19th edition.

7 T, T, F, F, F,

The luteal phase is always 14 days (i.e. progesterone peaks on day 21 of a 28-day cycle and day 28 of a 35-day cycle). If pregnancy occurs, serum beta-human chorionic gonadotrophin (sb-hCG) is produced by the trophoblast. This has a similar structure to LH. Both LH and sb-hCG cause the corpus luteum to mature (and not degenerate) in early pregnancy until the early placenta can produce progesterone, which is the predominant hormone of the luteal phase and early pregnancy. The granulosa cells have a yellow pigment called lutein, which is rich in cholesterol. Oestrogen and progesterone levels vary throughout the cycle. The perimenopause is associated with a high FSH level.

See Chapter 4, *Gynaecology by Ten Teachers*, 19th edition.

8   T, T, T, T, F

Diabetes is not associated with menstrual disorders. Non-insulin dependent diabetes mellitus (NIDDM) may be associated with polycystic ovary syndrome and thus anovulation which often causes oligomenorrhoea rather than menorrhagia.

See Chapter 5, *Gynaecology by Ten Teachers*, 19th edition.

9   T, F, T, F, T

The progesterone-only pill has a higher risk of ectopic pregnancy compared with the combined oral contraceptive pill and has a worse bleeding profile compared with the combined pill. As it does not inhibit ovulation in all women, it is quicker to effect resumption of ovulation after the progesterone-only pill has been stopped, compared with the combined oral contraceptive.

See Chapter 7, *Gynaecology by Ten Teachers*, 19th edition.

10   F, F, F, F, T

The main component of the Mirena IUS is levonorgestrel. The levonorgestrel intrauterine system (Mirena) is licensed currently for five years. Irregular heavy bleeding is a side effect associated with the copper coil; however, the Mirena is usually associated with reduction of menstrual loss. There is no increased risk of pelvic inflammatory disease with coil use; in fact, it is the same as with other contraceptive methods. The risk of infection is increased only at the time of insertion or removal.

See Chapter 7, *Gynaecology by Ten Teachers*, 19th edition.

11   T, T, F, F, F

The combined pill has a 12-hour window. Acute/severe liver disease is an absolute contraindication to COCP usage. The risk of VTE is 15 per 100 000 for second-generation users, 30 per 100 000 for third-generation users and 60 per 100 000 for pregnancy.

See Chapter 7, *Gynaecology by Ten Teachers*, 19th edition.

12   F, F, T, F, F

Investigations for infertility are expensive and some of them are invasive. Therefore, investigations should be directed towards each couple having gained an insight into the possible cause of infertility from the history. For example, a woman with a regular menstrual cycle may require only a mid-luteal progesterone to suggest ovulation occurs and does not need a full hormone profile. Further investigations are targeted according to the clinical picture. A low mid-luteal progesterone may confirm anovulation. A high progesterone of >30 nmol/L is certainly suggestive of but does not confirm ovulation. Ovulation can be truly confirmed only by serial scanning of ovarian follicles. However, in day-to-day use, a regular cycle and a progesterone level of >30 nmol/L are usually seen as indicative of ovulation. Full investigations for ovulatory disorders and male factor infertility are mandatory prior to embarking upon laparoscopy and tubal patency testing, as this procedure does have a morbidity associated with it. A hysterosalpingogram will gain information on tubal patency and uterine cavity outline; however, this does not give any indication of pelvic disease, such as previous pelvic infection or endometriosis. Laparoscopy allows the tubal patency to be assessed as well as staging degree of endometriosis or pelvic inflammatory disease. A normal semen analysis obtained after 3 days' abstention is sufficient to confirm a normal healthy population of sperm; however, a single suboptimal sample needs repeating to confirm oligospermia and further investigations are necessary until two suboptimal samples have been obtained. If a subsequent sample is normal, no further action is necessary.

See Chapter 8, *Gynaecology by Ten Teachers*, 19th edition.

13 T, T, T, F, F

Miscarriage is much more likely after the age of forty (30–40 per cent) compared with under the age of forty (6–10 per cent). The most common cause of spontaneous miscarriage is a spontaneous chromosomal defect.

See Chapter 9, *Gynaecology by Ten Teachers*, 19th edition.

14 F, T, T, T, T

Dermoid cysts often contain germ cells but NOT placental tissue.

See Chapter 9, *Gynaecology by Ten Teachers*, 19th edition.

15 F, F, T, T, F

The incidence of ectopic pregnancy is 22 per 1000 live births and 16 per 1000 pregnancies. Ectopic pregnancy is associated with chlamydial infection. Methotrexate is contraindicated if the mass is >2 cm in diameter.

See Chapter 9, *Gynaecology by Ten Teachers*, 19th edition.

16 T, F, F, T, T

Dermoid cysts are lined by either ectodermal tissue, such as skin, sebum or hair, or by endodermal tissue, such as bone or teeth. Typically, only 10 per cent of dermoids are bilateral.

See Chapter 12, *Gynaecology by Ten Teachers*, 19th edition.

17 T, F, T, T, T

Call–Exner bodies are pathognomonic of granulosa cell tumours.

See Chapter 12, *Gynaecology by Ten Teachers*, 19th edition.

18 F, F, T, T, F

Single cysts with no suspicious features tend not to be malignant. Multiple cysts located round the periphery with a dense stroma are pathognomonic of polycystic ovary syndrome. Calcification and fat are often suggestive of a dermoid cyst, which is benign.

See Chapter 12, *Gynaecology by Ten Teachers*, 19th edition.

19 T, F, F, F, F

AFP is elevated in endodermal yolk sac tumours and teratomas. Granulosa cell tumours have a raised inhibin marker. Epithelial cell tumours are associated with an elevated Ca 19-9. Choriocarcinoma and dysgerminoma are associated with an elevated beta-hCG.

See Chapter 12, *Gynaecology by Ten Teachers*, 19th edition.

20 F, T, F, T, F

See Chapter 14, *Gynaecology by Ten Teachers*, 19th edition.

21 T, T, F, F, T

Nulliparity and late menopause are risk factors for endometrial cancer along with ovarian tumour, previous pelvic irradiation and a family history of breast, ovary or colon cancer.

See Chapter 13, *Gynaecology by Ten Teachers*, 19th edition.

22 F, F, F, T, F

Carcinoma of the ovary is common in wealthy countries. It has a similar incidence to carcinoma of the endometrium but has a much greater mortality. The peak age is fifty to sixty; it is rare below thirty five years. The mainstay of treatment is surgery and chemotherapy with cisplatin and paclitaxol or carboplatin.

See Chapter 12, *Gynaecology by Ten Teachers*, 19th edition.

23 F, T, T, F, F

See Chapter 12, *Gynaecology by Ten Teachers*, 19th edition.

24 T, F, F, T, F

Late menopause is associated with ovarian cancer and the combined pill is protective against ovarian cancer, with a lifetime instance of four times less than those not using the pill. Implanon has no effect on the development of ovarian carcinoma.

See Chapter 12, *Gynaecology by Ten Teachers*, 19th edition.

25 T, T, T, T, T

CT allows visualization of local invasion and spread to lymph nodes. Barium enema and IVP evaluate tumour invasion into the rectum and descending colon and ureteric obstruction (although these are less commonly required). Ultrasound assesses the nature, size and location of the cyst along with CT. CA 125 is a non-specific tumour marker used to monitor treatment of ovarian cancer.

See Chapter 12, *Gynaecology by Ten Teachers*, 19th edition.

26 T, F, T, T, F

Cisplatin has a number of well-documented side effects, which include renal damage. However, the nephrotoxicity can be prevented by the use of vigorous diuresis. Cisplatin causes hypokalaemia. Cumulative dose-related neurotoxicity manifests as paraesthesia and ototoxicity.

See Chapter 12, *Gynaecology by Ten Teachers*, 19th edition.

27 T, F, F, T, F

Theca cell tumours and androblastomas are both sex-cord stroma tumours. Teratoma is a germ cell tumour.

See Chapter 12, *Gynaecology by Ten Teachers*, 19th edition.

28 F, F, T, T, F

The peak age of instance is below thirty years old. CA 125 is elevated in epithelial cell tumours, not dysgerminomas. Immature teratoma is malignant and the benign form is a mature teratoma, which is called a dermoid.

See Chapter 12, *Gynaecology by Ten Teachers*, 19th edition.

29 T, F, T, F, T

Although some systemic diseases such as diabetes are associated with pruritis vulvae, nephrotic syndrome is not. Vaginal discharge may be concurrent but is not a cause of pruritis vulvae.

See Chapter 15, *Gynaecology by Ten Teachers*, 19th edition.

30 F, T, T, T, F

Lichen sclerosis commonly affects the labia minora and the perianal region. Dark red and brown pigmentation is more suggestive of vulval intraepithelial neoplasia.

See Chapter 15, *Gynaecology by Ten Teachers*, 19th edition.

31 F, T, T, F, F

Primary syphilis causes vulval ulcers but tertiary syphilis causes neurosyphilis. HPV is not associated with vulval ulcers, but is associated with cervical intraepithelial neoplasia and cervical cancer. Ulcerative colitis does not cause benign vulval ulcers; however, Crohn's disease does.

See Chapter 15, Gynaecology by Ten Teachers, 19th edition.

32 F, F, T, T, F

The lower genital tract is lined by simple cuboidal epithelium in the pre-pubertal state and changes to stratified squamous under the influence of oestrogen. Oestrogen causes the vaginal pH to be reduced to around 3.5–4.5. Bacterial vaginosis is the most common cause of abnormal vaginal discharge in women of childbearing age.

See Chapter 15, *Gynaecology by Ten Teachers*, 19th edition.

33 F, T, F, F, F

Diagnosis of herpes simplex is made after collection of serum from vesicles. This is then analysed by electron microscopy or monolayer tissue culture. Reactivation arises in the dorsal root ganglia. Secondary infection in pregnancy does not require delivery by lower-segment Caesarean section as vertical transmission does not occur because the fetus develops passive immunity from maternal antibodies that cross the placenta. If there is a primary infection near term, delivery of the infant would be by Caesarean section. Antiviral treatment is not useful in established disease, as secondary infection usually resolves in the same time as viral treatment would work.

See Chapter 15, *Gynaecology by Ten Teachers*, 19th edition.

34 T, F, F, T, F

The most sensitive and specific test for syphilis is fluorescent treponemal antibody (FTA). This requires a skilled interpretation and most laboratories perform the *Treponema pallidum* haemagglutination assay (TPHA) or *Treponema pallidum* particle agglutination (TPPA) test instead. A non-specific test, such as the Venereal Disease Research Laboratory (VDRL) test, is often used in addition. Usually primary syphilis presents as a painless ulcer (chancre), with occasional regional lymph node enlargement. Treatment for syphilis is with simple penicillin.

See Chapter 15, *Gynaecology by Ten Teachers*, 19th edition.

35 F, T, T, F, T

Pelvic organ prolapse is predominantly found in multiparous women. The risk of prolapse increases with increasing parity. Pelvic organ prolapse affects around 2 per cent of nulliparous women and this suggests a congenital predisposition in these women despite them not undergoing childbirth. Epidural alone is not a risk factor for the development of prolapse; however, forceps macrosomia and malposition of the baby are associated with traumatic delivery and subsequent development of prolapse.

See Chapter 16, *Gynaecology by Ten Teachers*, 19th edition.

36 F, T, T, F, T

Large uterine fibroids and migraine with aura are relative contraindications to taking HRT.

See Chapter 18, *Gynaecology by Ten Teachers*, 19th edition.

37 T, T, T, T, F

Acne is a progestogen-related side effect of HRT.

See Chapter 18, *Gynaecology by Ten Teachers*, 19th edition.

38 F, F, T, T, F

The gestation should not exceed 24 weeks. The request for termination can be carried out only after two registered medical practitioners independently consider the effects of continuation of the pregnancy and feel that the woman has formed a judgement that termination is in her best interests. It is recommended that termination should be performed after 8 weeks' gestation, as the chance of missing fetal products and the pregnancy continuing are higher if the pregnancy is less than 8 weeks.

See Chapter 19, *Gynaecology by Ten Teachers*, 19th edition.

SINGLE BEST ANSWER QUESTIONS

QUESTIONS

Disorders of the menstrual cycle

1 NICE guidelines would recommend the best treatment of a forty-year-old woman with regular, heavy periods who smokes 20 cigarettes a day, has a BMI of 40 and has a normal-size, anteverted uterus on ultrasound scan and who is sexually active.
a) TAH.
b) TAH/BSO.
c) TCRE.
d) Combined oral contraceptive pill.
e) Mirena.

Genital infections in gynaecology

2 A patient presents with vulval itching, sore vagina and a profuse, white, curdy discharge with erythema and redness at the introitus. The likely diagnosis is:
a) Bacterial vaginosis.
b) Trichomonas vaginalis.
c) Candida.
d) Chlamydia.
e) HPV.

Fertility control, contraception and abortion

3 Choose from below the single best contraceptive method for a forty five-year-old woman with a BMI of 40, smoker with multiple fibroids, who is in a stable relationship, whose family is complete and who has had a peritonitis secondary to appendicitis in the past.
a) Combined oral contraceptive pill.

b) Laparoscopic clip sterilization.
c) Mirena.
d) Progesterone-only pill.
e) Hysteroscopic sterilization.

Subfertility

4   The hormone best used as a measurement of ovarian reserve is:
a) FSH.
b) Oestradiol.
c) LH.
d) Inhibin.
e) AMH.

Problems in early pregnancy

5   A nineteen year-old-girl is admitted with pelvic pain, a positive pregnancy test and a 3 cm viabe ectopic pregnancy seen in the right fallopian tube on ultrasound. She has already had a left saplingectomy for a previous ectopic. The best management would be:
a) Laparoscopic salpingectomy.
b) Laparoscopic salpingostomy.
c) Conservative management with serial βHCGs.
d) Laparotomy.
e) Methotrexate.

Benign diseases of the uterus and cervix

6   A twenty five-year-old girl presents with mid-cycle pain on a regular monthly basis. She is sexually active and does not take any contraception. The pain quickly resolves after 24 hours. She has a regular 28-day cycle. The likely cause of the pain is:
a) PID.
b) Endometriosis.
c) Mittelschmertz syndrome.
d) Adenomyosis.
e) Polycystic ovaries.

Endometriosis and adenomyosis

7   The most suitable treatment for a thirty four-year-old woman with minimal endometriosis on laparoscopy, who has been trying to conceive for two years and has pelvic pain, is:
a) Laser ablation to endometriosis/excision of the endometriosis.
b) GnRH analogues.
c) Danazol.
d) Progesterone.
e) Combined oral contraceptive pill.

Diseases of the ovary

8   A seventeen-year-old girl who is not sexually active presents with left iliac fossa pain. An ultrasound scan shows a 5 cm cyst on the left ovary which is complex in nature, with solid, calcified elements and fatty deposits noted on MRI. The likely diagnosis is:

a) Thecal luteal cyst.
b) Tubo-ovarian abscess.
c) Serous cystadenoma.
d) Fibroma.
e) Dermoid cyst.

Malignant disease of the uterus

9   The most appropriate treatment option for an eighty-year-old woman with a BMI of 25 presenting with post-menopausal bleeding and found to have Stage 1a endometrial adenocarcinoma on MRI and hysteroscopy is:

a)   Polypectomy and Mirena.
b)   TAH/BSO in a local centre.
c)   TAH/BSO in a cancer centre.
d)   TAH/BSO and radiotherapy.
e)   Radiotherapy alone.

Pre-malignant and malignant disease of the cervix

10   Management of a cervical smear showing moderate dyskaryosis is:
a) Repeat smear in six months.
b) HPV vaccination.
c) Colposcopy and biopsy.
d) LLETZ procedure.
e) Wertheim's hysterectomy.

Urogynaecology

11   The management of a thirty eight-year-old woman whose family is complete, with a BMI of 30 and who has urodynamically proven stress incontinence and a 4/5 score on the Oxford Grading Scale, would be:
a) Pelvic floor exercises.
b) Bladder neck injections.
c) Anterior repair.
d) Colposuspension.
e) TVT.

Pelvic organ prolapse

12   Management of an eighty nine-year-old woman with ischaemic heart disease who is not sexually active but presents with a procidentia of the uterus is:
a) Shelf pessary.

b) Pelvic floor exercises.
c) Vaginal hysterectomy.
d) Hysteroscopy.
e) Total vaginal mesh procedure.

Common gynaecological procedures

13 The procedure most suitable for the investigation of pelvic pain is:
a) Cystoscopy.
b) Hysteroscopy.
c) Hysterosalpingogram.
d) Laparoscopy.
e) Hysterectomy.

SBA ANSWERS

1 E

As this woman is sexually active and has a raised BMI and has not explored medical management, initially medical management would be advised before embarking on surgery such as a hysterectomy or endometrial resection or ablation. The combined oral contraceptive pill is a recognized medical management for menorrhagia but would be contraindicated in this woman as she has a raised BMI and is a smoker. As she has a normal-size cavity within the uterus, a Mirena would be the best choice. NICE guidelines would recommend Mirena in the initial management of menorrhagia and as the woman is under the age of forty five and has regular periods, she would not need endometrial sampling before trying the Mirena.
See Chapter 5, *Gynaecology by Ten Teachers*, 19th edition.

2 C

Bacterial vaginosis has a fishy, malodorous vaginal discharge and a creamy or greyish/white discharge without any itching or pain. Chlamydia is usually asymptomatic but may present with post-coital bleeding or a mild, mucopurulent cervical discharge. Trichomonas vaginalis presents with vulval soreness and itching and a foul-smelling vaginal discharge which is often frothy and yellowy/green. HPV presents with genital warts.
See Chapter 6, *Gynaecology by Ten Teachers*, 19th edition.

3 D

The combined oral contraceptive pill would be contraindicated if the woman has a BMI of 40. A Mirena is unlikely to fit within the uterine cavity as this woman has multiple fibroids. Sterilization is less attractive as she has had a previous laparotomy. The progesterone-only pill is as effective as the oral contraceptive pill in women over the age of forty. Hysteroscopic sterilization would be difficult in view of the multiple fibroids.
See Chapter 7, *Gynaecology by Ten Teachers*, 19th edition.

4 E

Anti-Müllerian hormone (AMH) levels can be measured in blood and are shown to be proportional to the number of small antral follicles. Serum AMH levels decrease with age and are undetectable in the post-menopausal period. AMH levels represent the quantity of the ovarian follicle pool and are a useful marker of ovarian reserve.
See Chapter 8, *Gynaecology by Ten Teachers*, 19th edition.

5 B

RCOG guidelines recommend laparoscopic salpingostomy in patients who have had a previous salpingectomy. This would at least retain some chance of subsequent fertility without the need for IVF. Conservative management and methotrexate are contraindicated as the pregnancy is too large and is viable on ultrasound scan. Laparotomy may be necessary but usually this can be treated with a laparoscopic approach.
See Chapter 9, *Gynaecology by Ten Teachers*, 19th edition.

6 C

As the pain is regular and occurs mid-cycle, this is most likely due to ovulation rather than endometriosis, which causes pre-menstrual pain and dyspareunia. Adenomyosis causes dysmenorrhoea. Polycystic ovary syndrome does not cause pelvic pain.
See Chapter 10, *Gynaecology by Ten Teachers*, 19th edition.

7 A

It has been recognized that subsequent fertility rates increase in patients with minimal endometriosis if this is excised or ablated using laser laparoscopy. The combined pill and GnRH analogues and danazol would all inhibit ovulation and therefore preclude the chances of pregnancy. Progesterone has not been shown to improve subsequent pregnancy rates.

See Chapter 11, *Gynaecology by Ten Teachers*, 19th edition.

8 E

Thecal luteal cysts are often complex in nature and have blood clots noted but no solid elements. The fibromas are solid elements but no calcified deposits. Tubo-ovarian abscesses usually have a mucopurulent complex nature. The fact that this cyst has calcified elements and fatty deposits on MRI is pathognomonic of a dermoid cyst.

See Chapter 12, *Gynaecology by Ten Teachers*, 19th edition.

9 B

If the adenocarcinoma is confined to the uterus and does not extend beyond 50 per cent of the myometrium, it is appropriate just to have a total abdominal hysterectomy and bilateral salpingo-oophorectomy with no subsequent radiotherapy. This can be performed in a local centre under current guidelines.

See Chapter 13, *Gynaecology by Ten Teachers*, 19th edition.

10 C

The smear test is a screening test and not a diagnostic test. As the smear shows moderate dyskaryosis, surveillance is no longer recommended and the patient requires colposcopic assessment. If, at colposcopic assessment, the colposcopic appearances are suggestive of CIN2, one could take a biopsy or perform a 'see and treat' LLETZ procedure. However, colposcopic assessment is mandatory before embarking straight for a LLETZ procedure.

See Chapter 14, *Gynaecology by Ten Teachers*, 19th edition.

11 E

As this patient has a 4/5 score on the Oxford Grading Scale, she has excellent pelvic floor contraction already and therefore would warrant surgical intervention. Anterior repair is not recognized as a suitable treatment for stress incontinence, only anterior compartment prolapse. Bladder neck injections can be useful but in a thirty eight year old, the longevity is very short lived. Colposuspension requires a laparotomy and has now been superceded by the tension-free vaginal tape procedure, which is recommended as gold standard under NICE guidelines.

See Chapter 16, *Gynaecology by Ten Teachers*, 19th edition.

12 A

As this lady is not sexually active and has numerous risk factors for surgery, a shelf pessary would be recommended in the first instance. Vaginal hysterectomy may be considered as a second-line treatment, but if she copes well with the pessary, this would negate the risk of surgery and anaesthesia. Total vaginal mesh is currently not recommended under NICE guidelines as first-line treatment for prolapse. Pelvic floor exercises have no role in Grade 2 or more prolapse.

See Chapter 17, *Gynaecology by Ten Teachers*, 19th edition.

13 D

Cystoscopy is useful for looking for conditions within the bladder. Hysteroscopy is the procedure to assess the uterine cavity for fibroids, investigation or post-menopausal bleeding, menorrhagia or fibroids. Hysterosalpingogram is useful to assess tubal patency in the investigation of the infertile couple. Hysterectomy would be a treatment rather than an investigative exploratory procedure.

See Appendix 1, *Gynaecology by Ten Teachers*, 19th edition.

SHORT ANSWER QUESTIONS

QUESTIONS

Normal and abnormal sexual development and puberty

1 **Write short notes on the salient features in the history and examination of a seventeen-year-old girl presenting with primary amenorrhoea.**

History

Developmental history: reflects sexual hormone production.
Presence/absence of cyclical symptoms: suggests ovarian function normal.
History of chronic illness: inhibits hypothalamic–pituitary–ovarian axis.
Excessive weight loss/eating disorder: inhibits hypothalamic–pituitary–ovarian axis.
Excessive exercise: inhibits hypothalamic–pituitary–ovarian axis.
Contraceptive history: menses on exogenous hormones may mask primary amenorrhoea.
Reproductive history: pregnancy is the most common cause of secondary amenorrhoea.
Menopausal symptoms and family history of premature menopause: a family history of premature ovarian failure may reflect a familial condition.
Medications: can inhibit hypothalamic–pituitary–ovarian axis, e.g. gonadotrophin-releasing hormone (GnRH) analogues.
Virilizing signs, galactorrhoea: suggests androgen-secreting tumour, congenital adrenal hyperplasia (CAH), prolactinoma.
Hirsutism, acne: may be suggestive of polycystic ovarian syndrome (PCOS). (12 marks)

Examination

Height: short stature may be associated with chromosomal abnormality, e.g. Turner's syndrome.
Weight/body mass index: polycystic ovary syndrome may be associated with raised BMI.
Secondary sexual characteristics/evidence of virilization: may reflect PCOS or androgen-secreting tumour.
Visual fields: homonymous hemianopia associated with pituitary tumour.
Pelvic examination: imperforate hymen, absent pelvic organs. (5 marks)

See Chapter 3, *Gynaecology by Ten Teachers,* 19th edition.

2 Write short notes on the five stages of puberty.

The events that occur in changes from a child to adult female usually occur in the following sequence:

1 Growth spurt.
2 Breast development.
3 Pubic hair growth.
4 Menstruation.
5 Axillary hair growth.

The above sequence of events occurs in around 70 per cent of girls but there may be minor differences in timing. Tanner has described pubertal development in five stages.   (3 marks)

The growth spurt starts at around eleven years of age owing to the effect of oestrogen and most girls have reached their final height by the age of 15 with the fusion of the femoral endplate.   (2 marks)

Breast bud development starts after the growth spurt in response to the production of oestradiol by the ovary. This is due to an increase in the production of GnRH from the pituitary gland. In initial breast development, the areola tissue appears more pronounced and then the breast tissue grows to become more confluent with the areola as it develops.   (2 marks)

Menarche is defined as the first menstrual period and occurs at any age between nine and seventeen years. Initially periods can be very irregular and it can take from five to eight years from the time of menarche for women to develop a regular cycle after full maturation of the hypothalamic–pituitary–ovarian axis.   (3 marks)

Pubic hair growth initially begins on the labia and then gradually extends over the mons pubis. Axillary hair growth is a late development.   (2 marks)

See Chapter 3, *Gynaecology by Ten Teachers*, 19th edition.

Disorders of the menstrual cycle

3 Write short notes on the history, examination and investigations for menorrhagia.

History
Last *menstrual period*. Cycle length and regularity of menses.
Duration of bleeding: number of days of heavy loss and lighter loss.
Passage of clots/flooding/number of sanitary protection used and how soaked.
Intermenstrual bleeding and post-coital bleeding.
Gynaecological history: pelvic inflammatory disease (associated with menorrhagia), smear history, contraception – intrauterine contraceptive device (IUCD) is associated with increased loss, or contraceptive pill, which regulates and usually decreases menstrual loss.
Symptoms of anaemia: lethargy, shortness of breath on exertion, syncope.   (4 marks)

Clinical examination
General:

- Endocrine disorders (hirsutism, striae, goitre, skin pigmentation, tremor).
- Secondary sexual characteristics.
- Signs of anaemia (tachycardia, pale sclerae).
- Liver disease, clotting disorder (bruising, petichiae).

Abdominal:

- Liver enlargement.
- Pelvic mass (suggestive of fibroids).

Vagina:

- Signs of trauma, infection.
- Visualize cervix for ectropion, malignancy.   (4 marks)

Investigations

NICE (National Institute for Health and Clinical Excellence) guidelines recommend a full blood count is needed to check for anaemia, platelet function.   (1 mark)

Thyroid function tests (TFTs): endocrine *only* if suspicion of thyroid disease.
Serum androgens: only if signs of hirsutism and acne.
Prolactin: only if oligomenorrhoea or lactation.
Coagulation screen: only if bruising, etc.
Urea and electrolytes (U&Es), liver function tests (LFTs): only if signs of renal/liver impairment.   (6 marks)

Pelvic ultrasound scan: to assess for fibroids if uterus enlarged or endometrial polyps, if intermenstrual bleeding.

Hysteroscopy/endometrial biopsy: NICE guidelines recommend hysteroscopy and endometrial biopsy in women over the age of forty five with menorrhagia or women under forty five with irregular bleeding to exclude malignancy and assess correlation of endometrial phase with cycle.   (2 marks)

See Chapter 5, *Gynaecology by Ten Teachers,* 19th edition.

Fertility control

4 Write short notes on the benefits, drawbacks, indications and contraindications for the combined oral contraceptive pill.

Benefits: reliable form of contraception (0.1–1 failure per 100 woman years), cycle control, reduces menorrhagia, recognized treatment of endometriosis.   (2 marks)

Drawbacks: as COCP inhibits ovulation, return to normal ovarian function may take twelve months after stopping; fluid retention; headaches; weight gain.   (2 marks)

Contraindications: certain forms of contraception would be contraindicated, especially the combined pill. The absolute contraindications to taking the combined oral contraceptive pill are:

- Circulatory disease, ischaemic heart disease, cerebrovascular accidents, significant hypertension, arterial or venous thrombosis, any acquired or inherited thrombotic tendency or any significant risk factors for cardiovascular disease.
- Acute or severe liver disease.
- Oestrogen-dependent neoplasms, particularly breast cancer.
- Focal migraine.   (4 marks)

The relative contraindications include:

- Generalized migraine.
- Long-term immobilization.
- Irregular vaginal bleeding, which has not had a diagnosis obtained.
- Less severe risk factors for cardiovascular disease, such as obesity, heavy smoking and diabetes.   (4 marks)

See Chapter 7, *Gynaecology by Ten Teachers,* 19th edition.

5 Outline the principal features that one would include in a consent form for women who are considering sterilization in an outpatient appointment.

Female sterilization is generally performed by occlusion of the Fallopian tubes. This is done using Filshie clips, plastic rings or with the use of excision and ligation of the tubes. The procedure is performed usually through laparoscopic surgery but can be performed as an open procedure, especially if concurrent surgery is occurring, e.g. Caesarean section. Hysteroscopic sterilization is becoming more widespread with promising results.

(2 marks)

It is advisable to warn the patient that the procedure should be considered permanent and irreversible. Reversal can be performed, but this is not provided under the NHS and no guarantees can be given about the success of reversal of sterilization.

(2 marks)

Failure of sterilization should be explained and the rate of 1 in 200 should be quoted. Failure rates rise due to either incomplete occlusion of the tubal lumen or recanalization of a previously appropriately occluded lumen. If sterilization fails owing to application of clips in the wrong structure, such as the round ligament, this is indefensible in court. It is, therefore, advisable to take photographs of the tubes once they are occluded at the time of surgery.

(3 marks)

The patient should be warned about the increased risk of ectopic pregnancy should they fall pregnant, although this is still very unlikely.

(1 mark)

If patients are using the combined oral contraceptive pill, their periods may be artificially light. Once they are sterilized, they will stop taking the combined pill and their periods will return to their physiological status. If the patient has had a history of menorrhagia, they should be warned that the chance of this recurring is high and alternative contraception, such as the Mirena, may be more appropriate.

(1 mark)

All other forms of contraception should be discussed with the patient, including male sterilization, which is safer, does not require a general anaesthetic and has a lower failure rate.

(1 mark)

See Chapter 7, *Gynaecology by Ten Teachers*, 19th edition.

Infertility

6 A couple attend the infertility clinic for the first time having been trying to conceive a pregnancy for the last twelve months of unprotected intercourse. What are the salient points in the history?

Maternal age: rates of conception decline rapidly after the age of 35.

(1 mark)

Parity and gravidity: ages and modes of delivery of previous pregnancies.

(2 marks)

Menstrual cycle: regularity of menstrual cycle suggests but does not confirm ovulation; oligomenorrhoea or amenorrhoea may be suggestive of an ovulatory disorder.

(1 mark)

Contraception: previous contraception is important, as some contraceptives, such as the Depo, can have a prolonged effect.

(1 mark)

Disorders suggestive of a general endocrine problem: one should list in the history symptoms that may suggest an endocrine disorder that can affect ovulation.

(1 mark)

Tubal disease: one should look in the history for risk factors for tubal disease, such as a history of sexually transmitted diseases/PID, pelvic abscesses, pelvic or abdominal surgery, tubal surgery and previous ectopic pregnancies.

(2 marks)

General history: one should ask about smear history, rubella status and blood group, if known, as well as discussing pre-conceptual folic acid, which should be taken for three months peri-conception. On general examination, one should look for signs of raised BMI, hirsutism and other endocrine disorders, and secondary sexual characteristics. On abdominal examination, one should inspect for signs of abdominal/pelvic surgery and vaginal examination should be performed. Swabs should be taken for chlamydia, gonorrhoea and other sexually transmitted diseases, and a smear should be obtained if patient has not had one as part of the normal recall process.   (4 marks)

History and examination of male partner: this is essential. One should note age, history of any children in this relationship or other relationships, smoking, alcohol use and occupation. It is important to enquire about testicular trauma, undescended testes, mumps and sexually transmitted diseases. On examination, one should assess the size of each testis, check for varicoceles and descent, and note secondary sexual characteristics. One should also discuss quite openly the couple's frequency and timing of coitus to ensure this is occurring during the fertile time of the woman's cycle (i.e. 14 days prior to menstrual period).   (4 marks)

See Chapter 8, *Gynaecology by Ten Teachers*, 19th edition.

Disorders of early pregnancy

7 Write short notes on threatened miscarriage, silent miscarriage and incomplete miscarriage.

Threatened miscarriage
This is defined as bleeding in early pregnancy of <24 weeks' gestation. The patient presents with vaginal bleeding that may be associated with suprapubic pain. On vaginal examination, the cervical os is closed. Ultrasound demonstrates a gestational sac with a fetal pole and the fetal heart is seen. There may or may not be an intrauterine haematoma present.   (3 marks)

Silent miscarriage
Patients may present either with minimal bleeding, old blood loss or no bleeding at all. Sometimes the diagnosis is made incidentally at ultrasound scan when patients come for a routine 12-week or 20-week scan. The diagnosis is confirmed if ultrasound shows an embryo of <20 weeks with no fetal heart and no signs of expulsion. Alternatively, a gestation sac of 0.20 mm and no embryo, or a fetal pole of 0.6 mm with no fetal heart seen, would be classified as a missed miscarriage. Management can be either medically induced miscarriage or surgical evacuation.   (3 marks)

Incomplete miscarriage
Patients usually present with heavy bleeding and cramping pain, and have partial expulsion of the products of conception. On speculum examination, if the cervical os is open, it is termed an 'inevitable miscarriage'. A transvaginal scan will show products of conception within the uterine cavity. The management can be either expectant, surgical evacuation or medical, and depends on the size of the products of conception within the uterine cavity. As a general rule, if the products of conception are 0.50 mm, surgical or medical evacuation would be recommended.   (4 marks)

See Chapter 9, *Gynaecology by Ten Teachers*, 19th edition.

8 Write short notes on the diagnosis and management of ectopic pregnancy.

Clinical presentation
The majority of patients present with abdominal pain ± vaginal bleeding. Occasionally, patients have shoulder-tip pain indicative of free blood in abdominal cavity. Bimanual examination reveals tenderness in the fornices ± cervical excitation.   (3 marks)

Investigation
The following are useful: pulse, temperature, blood pressure, haemoglobin, HCG, transvaginal ultrasound scan.
                                                                                                                            (2 marks)

Management

Ectopic pregnancies can be managed expectantly. This is suitable only for patients who are haemodynamically stable and asymptomatic. Medical management involves treatment with methotrexate. The following are reasonable indications:

a) Cornual pregnancy.
b) Trophoblastic disease.
c) Patient with one Fallopian tube and fertility is desired.
d) Patient who refuses surgery or on whom risks of surgery are too high.

Surgical management is usually by laparoscopy or laparotomy. Laparoscopic approach has less blood loss and shorter operating time. At laparoscopy, one can perform either salpingectomy or salpingostomy.   (4 marks)

See Chapter 9, *Gynaecology by Ten Teachers*, 19th edition.

Benign diseases of the uterus and cervix

9 Write short notes on the principles of a screening programme.

There are 10 principles of screening that are now adopted by the World Health Organization.

1 The condition should be an important health problem.   (1 mark)
2 There should be a recognizable latent or early symptomatic stage.   (1 mark)
3 The natural history of the condition, including development from latent to declared disease, should be adequately understood.   (1 mark)
4 There should be an accepted treatment for patients with recognized disease and early intervention will alter prognosis compared with treatment of later manifested disease.   (1 mark)
5 There should be a suitable test or examination.   (1 mark)
6 The test should be acceptable to the population.   (1 mark)
7 There should be an agreed policy on whom to treat as patients.   (1 mark)
8 Facilities for diagnosis and treatment should be available.   (1 mark)
9 The cost of screening (including diagnosis and treatment of patients diagnosed should be economically balanced in relation to possible expenditure to medical care of patients with declared disease.   (1 mark)
10 Screening should be a continuing process and not a 'once and for all' project.   (1 mark)

See Chapter 10, *Gynaecology by Ten Teachers*, 19th edition.

Endometriosis and adenomyosis

10 Outline the four theories for the pathophysiology of endometriosis.

1 *Menstrual regurgitation and implantation.* One theory is that endometriosis occurs as a result of retrograde menstruation and that implantation of endometrial glands and tissue occurs into the peritoneal surface. This has been shown to occur in experimental models.   (2 marks)
2 *Coelomic epithelium transformation.* Another theory is that peritoneal cells and cells in the ovary which are derived from the Müllerian duct undergo dedifferentiation back to their primitive origin and then transform into endometrial cells. It is not yet known what might stimulate this dedifferentiation.
                                                                                                   (2 marks)
3 *Genetic and immunological factors.* Some women of certain genetic/immunological predisposition may possess factors that render them susceptible to the development of endometriosis. This is substantiated by a familial tendency as well as racial tendencies.   (2 marks)

4 *Vascular lymphatic spread.* Occasionally endometriosis can be found inside and outside the peritoneal cavity, such as skin, kidney and lung. This may occur due to embolization of endometrial tissue via vascular lymphatic channels or at surgery.   (2 marks)

See Chapter 11, *Gynaecology by Ten Teachers*, 19th edition.

11 Write short notes on the initial investigation and management of a patient with suspected endometriosis.

History

The salient features include dysmenorrhoea, the demonstration of cyclical pelvic pain, deep dyspareunia, a history of sub-fertility or infertility. Bladder symptoms may include cyclical haematuria or ureteric obstruction, and bowel symptoms may include cyclical rectal bleeding or pain on defecation.   (3 marks)

Examination

Pain in the pouch of Douglas provoked by palpation over the rectovaginal septum and uterosacral ligaments. It is sometimes possible to palpate nodules of endometriosis on rectovaginal examination. Bidigital examination may help palpate any pelvic masses such as endometriomas.   (3 marks)

Differential diagnoses

Adenomyosis, pelvic inflammatory disease or bowel pathology (irritable bowel syndrome).   (1 mark)

Investigations

Ultrasound scan to exclude any endometriomas. A CA 125 is of little clinical use but may be slightly raised in endometriosis. A diagnostic laparoscopy with or without tubal patency testing will confirm a diagnosis of endometriosis, and endometrial explants can be seen within the peritoneal cavity.   (4 marks)

See Chapter 11, *Gynaecology by Ten Teachers*, 19th edition.

12 Write short notes on the differences in epidemiology, symptomatology, investigation and treatment of endometriosis and adenomyosis.

Adenomyosis tends to affect women between the ages of thirty and forty, whereas endometriosis tends to affect women in their late twenties and thirties.   (2 marks)

Women with adenomyosis present with increasingly severe secondary spasmodic dysmenorrhoea and increased menorrhagia. On examination, they tend to have a tender uterus, particularly pre-menstrually. In women with an endometrioma, tenderness is usually elicited in the pouch of Douglas, rectovaginal septum and adnexae.   (3 marks)

The diagnosis of adenomyosis can sometimes be suspected on ultrasound if there is asymmetrical irregular echogenicity within the myometrium. Magnetic resonance imaging provides further enhanced images and is the investigation of choice. If the patient has endometriosis, ultrasound may demonstrate the presence of endometriomas. The diagnosis of adenomyosis can only truly be made at hysterectomy as it is an histological finding.   (3 marks)

Endometriosis can be treated by simple analgesia. Inhibition of ovulation using the combined oral contraceptive pill and GnRH analogues can give symptomatic relief. Ablation, resection or total abdominal hysterectomy and bilateral salpingo-oophorectomy are more definitive. Adenomyosis is treated definitively by hysterectomy.   (2 marks)

See Chapter 11, *Gynaecology by Ten Teachers*, 19th edition.

Benign diseases of the ovary

13 Outline the different strategies for the management of a single 4 cm ovarian cyst in the pre-menopausal, pregnant and post-menopausal woman.

Pre-menopausal
Cysts on the ovary can be physiological, benign or malignant. Physiological cysts usually measure less than 40 cm. Physiological cysts are more common in this age group. An ultrasound and CA 125 may help differentiate whether the cyst is sinister or pathological. Sinister findings would be septae, solid elements or large cysts. If the cyst appears suspicious and may or may not have elevated tumour markers, discussion at a multidisciplinary meeting is advisable to decide on whether surgery is indicated and what procedure would be most appropriate. If the cyst is symptomatic (painful), treatment either by laparoscopy or laparotomy would be warranted.
(4 marks)

Pregnant
Cysts are often found asymptomatically at ultrasound, at antenatal clinic or at Caesarean section. The risk of torsion is increased in pregnancy due to the movement of the pelvic organs out of the pelvis as the gravid uterus grows. Ultrasound monitoring during each trimester is sufficient provided the patient remains asymptomatic. Surgery should be avoided until 14 weeks to reduce the risk of miscarriage and intervention with a corpus luteum, which should have regressed by 12 weeks. Surgery is usually contemplated if the patient's symptoms are serious, such as significant pain, cyst rupture and significant bleeding or torsion. Tocolysis is often used at the time of surgery to reduce the risk of miscarriage and preterm labour.
(4 marks)

Post-menopausal
Physiological cysts on the ovary are unlikely in the post-menopause but can still be found. Evaluation of the cyst using ultrasound, CA 125, Doppler and the patient's age can be entered into an equation to give a risk of malignancy (relative malignancy index). If the risk of malignancy score is low and the patient is asymptomatic, patients can be left alone with no further follow-up. If the malignancy score is high, referral and discussion through a multidisciplinary team meeting should be arranged, with possible subsequent hysterectomy and bi-lateral oopherectomy if malignancy is suspected.
(4 marks)

See Chapter 12, *Gynaecology by Ten Teachers*, 19th edition.

14 A forty-year-old patient presents with a history of ovarian cysts. She is admitted with acute abdominal pain after 2 weeks of pelvic discomfort and urinary frequency. On examination, there is a mass palpable arising out of the pelvis. What is the differential diagnosis? What are the salient features in the history and examination, and how would you investigate the patient?
The most likely differential diagnoses would include a benign ovarian cyst, cyst rupture or torsion, urinary retention, fibroids (possibly degenerating). Other less likely diagnoses would include appendicitis with appendix abscess, PID/pyo-/hydrosalpinx.
(3 marks)

Salient features in the history would include the last menstrual period (if late exclude pregnancy) and cycle length, contraception, previous ovarian cysts or fibroids, sexual history, pain (whether this was associated with vomiting or rigors as this may be suggestive of appendicitis/torsion/PID). Shoulder-tip pain or bleeding may be indicative of ectopic pregnancy.
(3 marks)

On ultrasound, benign cysts tend to be large and unilocular simple cysts, whereas malignant tumours have septae, are often solid or semisolid, and are larger. A raised CA 125 is strongly suggestive of ovarian carcinoma, but can also be mildly elevated in endometriosis and pelvic inflammatory disease. If ultrasound and CA 125 suggest a malignancy, a CT scan is mandatory to evaluate further the nature of the cyst as well as nodal spread. (4 marks)

See Chapter 12, *Gynaecology by Ten Teachers*, 19th edition.

Malignant disease of the uterus and cervix

15 Write short notes on the risk factors, investigation and management of patients with post-menopausal bleeding.

The likely differential diagnoses include atrophic vaginal tissues, endometrial polyp or endometrial hyperplasia/adenocarcinoma. (2 marks)

Risk factors for endometrial hyperplasia/adenocarcinoma are diabetes, obesity, PCOS, unopposed oestrogen.

Initial investigations involve examination of the lower genital tract looking for atrophic tissues, as well as bimanual examination to assess uterine size and feel for parametrial thickening, which would be suggestive of malignancy. (3 marks)

Pelvic ultrasound scan is useful to measure endometrial thickness and, if this is <4 mm, the patient can be reassured that the risk of malignancy is almost zero, providing they have had only a single episode of post-menopausal bleeding. In this instance, the patients can be discharged but should reattend if they have any further bleeding. Outpatient hysteroscopy and Pipelle aspiration of the endometrium is useful if the endometrial thickness is >4 mm. Rigid saline hysteroscopy occasionally needs to be performed under general anaesthesia for patients who cannot tolerate outpatient hysteroscopy. Another indication for rigid saline hysteroscopy would be if the patient has findings on ultrasound suggestive of a polyp, which cannot be removed in the outpatient setting. (3 marks)

Treatment would depend on the cause. If the patient has atrophic tissues, topical oestrogens are appropriate. A polypectomy can be performed if there is a single polyp that is benign. The mainstay of treatment for endometrial carcinoma is total abdominal hysterectomy and bilateral salpingo-oophorectomy with or without post-operative radiotherapy. Bilateral pelvic lymph nodes and para-aortic node sampling is often performed if there are concerns regarding malignancy. (3 marks)

See Chapters 13 and 14, *Gynaecology by Ten Teachers*, 19th edition.

Carcinoma of the ovary and Fallopian tube

16 Write short notes on the classification of epithelioid tumours of the ovary.

Epithelioid tumours can be classified into serous, mucinous, endometrioid, clear cell, Brenner and undifferentiated tumours. (1 mark)

The majority of serous tumours have solid and cystic elements, are often bilateral and have psammoma bodies present on histology. (2 marks)

Mucinous tumours account for 10 per cent of the malignant tumours of the ovary. They are usually multilocular thin-walled cysts with a smooth surface full of mucinous fluid. Mucinous cysts often have exceedingly large dimensions. (2 marks)

Endometrioid tumours resemble the endometrium of the uterus in histology. They are often cystic unilocular cysts containing turbid, brown fluid. A total of 15 per cent are associated with an endometrial cancer of the uterus.   (2 marks)

Clear cell tumours are the least common epithelial tumours and often coexist with endometrioid tumours or endometriosis.   (2 marks)

Borderline tumours account for 10 per cent of ovarian tumours. They are usually confined to the ovary and have a better prognosis.   (1 mark)

See Chapter 12, *Gynaecology by Ten Teachers*, 19th edition.

Infections in gynaecology

17 Write short notes on candida, bacterial vaginosis and trichomoniasis vaginalis.

Candida

This is a fungal infection usually caused by the *Candida albicans* organism in 80 per cent of women. It is not sexually transmitted and women usually present with an itchy, sore vagina and vulva, and a curdy white discharge. Topical treatment is usually sufficient with clotrimazole 500 mg, although oral fluconazole is an alternative.   (3 marks)

Bacterial vaginosis

This is not a sexually transmitted disease. It is typically caused by anaerobic organisms, such as *Gardnerella vaginalis, Bacteroides, Mobiluncus* and *Micoplasma spp*. Women typically present with an offensive fishy, frothy discharge. Diagnosis is made on composite Ansel criteria. These criteria are: (1) a pH of 4.5; (2) a fishy smell on the application of potassium hydrochloride; (3) 'clue' cells on microscopy. It is treated with either oral or topical metronidazole. There is an increased risk of second trimester miscarriage and preterm labour, and women with a history of this should be screened and treated for the organisms.   (4 marks)

Trichomoniasis vaginalis

This is a sexually transmitted disease, the incidence of which is falling in the UK. Women usually present with a yellow or green discharge. Examination of the cervix shows multiple punctate haemorrhages, which give the characteristic 'strawberry' cervix. The diagnosis is made after culturing organisms in Fireberg Whittington medium. The treatment of choice is metronidazole.   (3 marks)

See Chapter 6, *Gynaecology by Ten Teachers*, 19th edition.

Urogynaecology

18 Write short notes on the investigation and management of an overactive bladder.
Detrusor overactivity is a urodynamics observation characterized by involuntary detrusor contractions during the filling phase, which may be spontaneous or provoked.   (1 mark)

Patients usually present with symptoms of urgency, frequency and nocturia (OAB syndrome dry). Patients may also complain of urgency incontinence – overactive bladder syndrome (OAB syndrome wet).   (1 mark)

Conservative management would include lifestyle changes such as cutting out caffeine, bladder retraining, biofeedback, pelvic floor exercises.   (2 marks)

Medical treatments involve the use of anticholinergics. The main side effects include dry mouth, constipation and central nervous system side effects.   (2 marks)

Intradetrusor injection with botulin toxin (Botox) has been shown to help with both neurogenic and idiopathic detrusor overactivity. However, 20 per cent of patients may fail to void after botulinum injection and have to intermittently self-catheterize.   (2 marks)

Sacral nerve stimulation is an alternative therapy, maybe either with an in-dwelling, permanent implant or transdermal patch or percutaneous tibial nerve stimulation.   (2 marks)

See Chapter 16, *Gynaecology by Ten Teachers*, 19th edition.

The menopause

19 Write short notes on the effects the menopause and its hypo-oestrogenic state have on the female physiology.
Symptoms of the menopause are usually stimulated by a fall in circulating oestrogen and may occur prior to the absolute level defined at the post-menopause of <100 pmol/L. Symptoms include tiredness, hot flushes, night sweats, insomnia, vaginal dryness and urinary frequency, recurrent urinary tract infections and dyspareunia.   (3 marks)

Various physiological changes occur and these can affect different systems of the body, predominantly the skeletal and cardiovascular systems. Oestrogen acts to prevent bone turnover by balancing the equilibrium between bone resorption and bone formation. A low circulating oestrogen is associated with a greater bone resorption rate over bone formation in the trabecular bone. Trabecular bone has a higher surface area, thus post-menopausal women are at particular risk of osteopaenia and osteoporosis. They are also at higher risk of traumatic fractures, typically of the distal radius and neck of femur.   (3 marks)

The cardiovascular system is the second major physiological system affected in the post-menopausal period and the incidence of myocardial infarction rises significantly at this time. A hypo-oestrogenic state is associated with significant changes in the lipid profile that predisposes women to atheroma. These include raised total cholesterol, lower HDL cholesterol and a high LDL (low-density lipoprotein). Triglycerides remain at similar levels to those in the pre-menopausal state. Oestrogen also causes vasoconstriction, owing to reduction in the production of nitrogen synthase. Large randomized controlled trials have shown no benefit and possibly a deleterious effect on the cardiovascular system with the administration of hormone replacement therapy. Therefore it is not recommended to start this as a treatment for or prevention of cardiovascular disease.   (4 marks)

See Chapter 18, *Gynaecology by Ten Teachers*, 19th edition.

OBJECTIVE STRUCTURED CLINICAL EXAMINATION QUESTIONS

QUESTIONS

1 History and examination

Outline a format for a gynaecological history, including headings and subheadings.

2 History and examination

Name the two devices seen in Figures 10.1 and 10.2 and outline the patient's position for examination with each, along with their clinical applications.

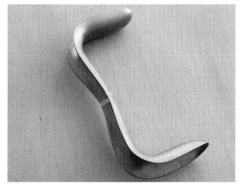

Figure 10.1

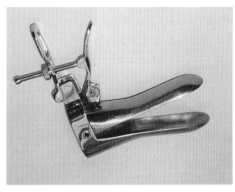

Figure 10.2

3 Embryology, anatomy and physiology

Label the diagrams below of the human female pelvis (Figures 10.3 and 10.4).

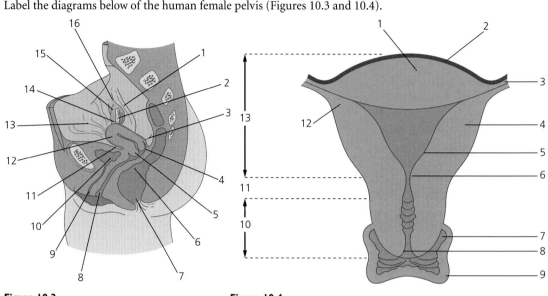

Figure 10.3   **Figure 10.4**

4 Normal and abnormal sexual development and puberty

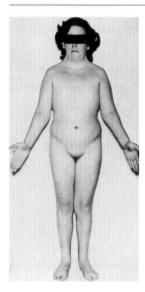

Figure 10.5

a) What clinical condition is demonstrated in Figure 10.5?
b) What is the typical karyotype?
c) List the typical clinical features.
d) What is the typical hormone profile of this patient?
e) What is the macroscopic appearance of the ovaries at laparotomy for this condition?
f) What are the two phases of treatment for this patient?

5 The normal menstrual cycle

Draw the menstrual cycle, outlining changes in the hypothalamic, pituitary and ovarian hormone levels as well as the changes that occur in the ovary and endometrium.

6 The normal menstrual cycle

Label these histology sections of endometrium (Figure 10.6a and b) and match the features listed below with each phase.

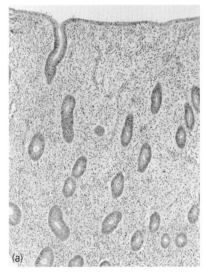

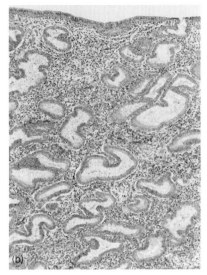

Figure 10.6(a)   **Figure 10.6(b)**

Phase:
- Follicular phase.
- Secretory phase.
- Luteal phase.
- Proliferative phase.

Characteristics:

- Stromal oedema and glandular growth.
- Glandular and stromal proliferation.
- Pre-ovulation.
- Post-ovulation.
- Progesterone predominates.
- Oestrogen predominates.

7 Fertility control

List the various methods of contraception along with their failure rate per 100 per women years.

8 Fertility control (role play)

A sixteen-year-old girl attends a clinic having forgotten to take her combined oral contraceptive pill. How would you counsel her?

9 Fertility control

List the modes of action of the following contraceptives:

- Combined oral contraceptive pill.
- Progesterone-only pill.
- Depo.
- Intrauterine device (IUD).
- Intrauterine system (IUS).
- Condoms.
- Natural family planning.
- Female sterilization.
- Male sterilization.

10 Infertility (role play)

A couple are referred to the infertility clinic having tried to conceive a pregnancy after 2 years of unprotected intercourse. Mrs Smith is twenty nine, has irregular periods (two to three per year), she weighs 16 stone, has significant acne and facial hair. She has no history of pelvic surgery or pelvic infections. Mr Smith has a normal semen analysis and has children from a previous relationship. The investigations from the female partner are as follows:

Table 10.1	
Day 2 luteinizing hormone	12 u/L
Follicle-stimulating hormone	4 u/L
Prolactin	Normal
Sex hormone binding globulin	Reduced
Testosterone	High
Day 24 progesterone	4 nmol/L

A hysterosalpingogram demonstrates bilateral tubal patency with a normal uterine cavity. The ultrasound scan of Mrs Smith's ovaries is shown in Figure 10.7.

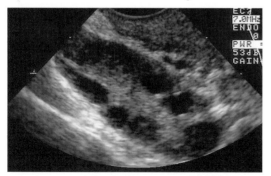

Figure 10.7

a) What is the likely diagnosis?
b) How would you initially try to counsel and manage this patient?

11 Disorders of early pregnancy

A seventeen-year-old woman presents to the early pregnancy assessment unit complaining of 7 weeks' amenorrhoea, nausea and vomiting, breast tenderness, moderate bleeding and intermittent abdominal pain.

a) On examination, she has a normal pulse and blood pressure, there are no signs of peripheral shutdown, she has no adnexal tenderness, the cervix is closed and non-tender. Urinary pregnancy test is positive. What are the possible diagnoses?

b) A transvaginal scan demonstrates a gestation sac of 30 mm, a yolk sac, a fetal pole, and a fetal heart is clearly seen beating. A large haematoma of 40 mm is seen adjacent to the gestation sac. A corpus luteum was noted on the right ovary measuring 25 mm and the left ovary was normal. There was no free fluid or any other adnexal mass noted. What is the diagnosis and your initial management?

c) Two weeks later, the woman returns for a repeat scan as she has experienced further bleeding. On ultrasound, the gestation sac measures 29 mm, the yoke sac is seen, but no fetal heart movements are seen. What would you do next?

12 Benign diseases of the uterus and cervix

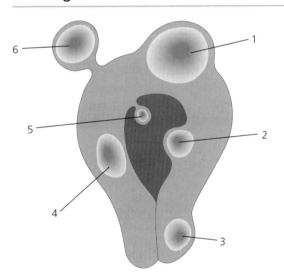

Figure 10.8

a) Label Figure 10.8.
b) What are the typical clinical presentations?
c) What are the different types of degeneration?

13 Benign diseases of the uterus and cervix

A thirty four-year-old nulliparous woman from Ghana is referred by her GP complaining of menorrhagia, dysmenorrhoea, urinary frequency, right loin pain and constipation. On examination, she is normotensive with a pulse of 98 beats per minute, she has pale sclerae and she has a pelvic mass extending above the umbilicus. Her last menstrual period was a week ago, was extremely heavy and has just stopped.

a) What are the possible diagnoses?
b) What investigations would you perform and why?
c) An ultrasound scan shows a large, fundal, subserous fibroid and several submucous fibroids, the largest being 3 cm in diameter. They do not appear to impinge on the uterine cavity. The renal ultrasound scan shows normal renal tracts with no evidence of obstruction. A mid-stream urine confirms that the patient had a

urinary tract infection; this was treated and her loin pain improved. Haemoglobin was low, with a low mean corpuscular volume. What options would you offer to the patient?

14 Pre-malignant and malignant diseases of the uterus and cervix

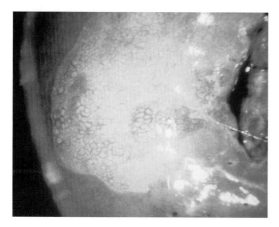

Figure 10.9

a) What is this image from?
b) What are the typical features seen during this investigation?
c) What is the likely diagnosis?
d) What is the treatment for this condition?
e) What is the common cause of this condition?
f) Why is it important to treat this?
g) What is the follow-up for these patients?

15 Infections in gynaecology

A twenty-year-old woman presents with a 3-day history of pelvic pain, vaginal discharge and fever. She had unprotected intercourse 10 days ago with her new partner. On examination, she has cervical excitation, a mucopurulent discharge and tenderness in both adnexae. Figure 10.10 illustrates findings at laparoscopy.

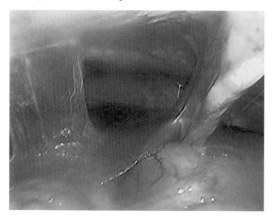

Figure 10.10

a) What is this condition called?
b) What is the most common causative organism?

c) What are the other possible causes?
d) What cells do the main causative organisms colonize?
e) What tests are used to make the diagnosis?
f) What are the most common treatments?
g) What other precautions have to be taken?
h) What are the risks associated with subsequent pregnancy?

16 Infections in gynaecology

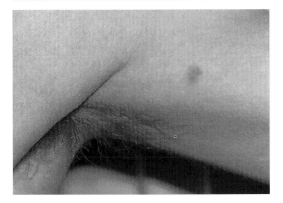

Figure 10.11

a) What is seen in the photograph above?
b) What condition is this associated with and what is the causative organism?
c) What is the natural history of infection?
d) How is it transmitted?
e) What type of organism is the virus?
f) How does this replicate?
g) How is the diagnosis made and how is the disease monitored?
h) What is the treatment of choice?

17 Urogynaecology

This is a urinary diary of an eighty-year-old woman who complains of urinary incontinence.

	Day 1		Day 2		Day 3	
Time	**Volume in (mL)**	**Urine out (mL)**	**Volume in (mL)**	**Urine out (mL)**	**Volume in (mL)**	**Urine out (mL)**
7 am		250		200		220
8 am	300		330		330	100
9 am		100		150		
10 am	200	75		100		100
11 am			330		200	50
12 pm		100		100		50
1 pm		100		75		

Table 10.2

(Continued)

Table 10.2 (Continued)

Time	Day 1 Volume in (mL)	Day 1 Urine out (mL)	Day 2 Volume in (mL)	Day 2 Urine out (mL)	Day 3 Volume in (mL)	Day 3 Urine out (mL)
2 pm	175		200			100
3 pm		100		75	450	
4 pm		75		100		75
5 pm						50
6 pm	400	50	450	100		50
7 pm				50	450	
8 pm	100	100	330	50		100
9 pm	200	75		50		100
10 pm			330		300	
11 pm			100			100
12 am		100				
1 am				100		100
2 am		100				100
3 am		100		100		
4 am						100
5 am				100		
6 am						

a) What is this patient's bladder functional capacity?
b) What is the patient's daytime frequency?
c) What is the patient's night-time frequency?
d) What are the possible diagnoses?

The patient complains of leakage with coughing as well as urgency, frequency, nocturia and occasional urge incontinence. Formal cystometry is performed and the results are given below.

Table 10.3

Maximum capacity	280 mL
First sensation	80 mL
First urgency	90 mL
Maximum detrusor pressure	A peak up to 20 cm of water was noted after a cough
Voided volume	320 mL
Flow rate	20 mL/second
Detrusor pressure at peak flow	60 cm of water

a) What is the diagnosis?
b) This woman had cystometry due to multiple mixed symptoms. What are the other indications for urodynamics?

18 Urogynaecology

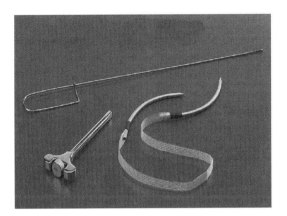

Figure 10.12

a) What does the picture above show?
b) What condition is it used to treat?
c) What was the traditional treatment for this condition?
d) What are the main benefits and morbidities associated with the traditional procedure?
e) What are the advantages of the above procedure versus the traditional procedure?

19 Uterovaginal prolapse

a) Label the diagram below.
b) Describe the three mechanisms of support for pelvic organs.

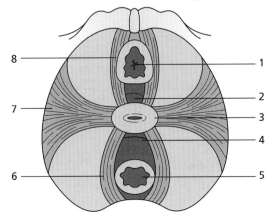

Figure 10.13

20 Uterovaginal prolapse

Classification and grading of prolapse

a) Complete the following table:

Table 10.4		
Compartment	**Organ**	**Nomenclature of prolapse**
Anterior	1	7
	2	8
Posterior	3	9
	4	10
Apex	5	11
	6	12

b) Describe the grading system with regards to primary, secondary and tertiary prolapse.

21 The menopause (role play)

A fifty-year-old woman with no significant obstetric history and no previous operations attends your clinic requesting hormone replacement therapy. She has been amenorrhoeic for nine months and suffers from hot flushes.

Conduct a consultation on how you would counsel the patient, highlighting the following:

a) Contraindications to HRT.
b) Modes of delivery for HRT.
c) Sites of action of oestrogen.
d) When progesterone should be administered.
e) The two types of oestrogen and progesterone regimen, and when they should be used.

22 Common gynaecological procedures

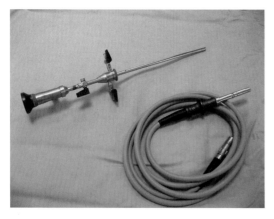

a) What is shown in Figure 10.14?
b) List indications for the use of this procedure.
c) List the complications of this procedure.

Figure 10.14

23 Common gynaecological procedures

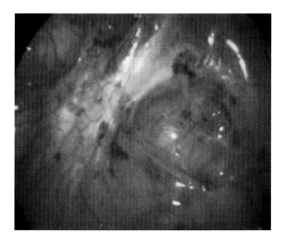

a) What is the image seen in the photograph?
b) What is the instrument used to provide this image?
c) What are the clinical indications for this procedure?
d) What are the complications of the procedure?

OSCE ANSWERS

1 History and examination

Name, age, occupation
Main presenting complaint

History of presenting complaint

- Menstrual history:
  - Pattern of bleeding (regular/irregular)
  - Amount of loss (clots/flooding/sanitary protection)
- Intermenstrual bleeding
- Pelvic pain: ? related to cycle, site and nature, radiation
- Dyspareunia (superficial/deep)
- Vaginal discharge
- Fertility history/urogynaecology questions

Menstrual cycle

- Menarche
- Number of days bleeding/number of days between periods
- First day of last menstrual period

Gynaecological history

- Previous investigations and procedures
- Smear history

Obstetric history

- Number of previous pregnancies
- Number of previous live births, stillbirths, miscarriages, terminations
- Birthweights and mode of delivery of live births

Sexual and contraceptive history

- Dyspareunia
- Sexually transmitted diseases
- Contraception

Medical history/drug history and allergies Social history

- Occupation
- Smoking and alcohol intake

Systemic enquiry

2 History and examination

Figure 10.1: Sim's speculum. The patient lies in the left lateral position; it is used to inspect the vault and anterior vaginal wall.

Figure 10.2: Cusco's (bivalve) speculum. The patient lies in the lithotomy position; it is used to inspect the exposed cervix.

3 Embryology, anatomy and physiology

Figure 10.3: 1, Right ureter; 2, ovary; 3, rectouterine fold; 4, posterior fornix; 5, cervix uteri; 6, rectal ampulla; 7, anal canal; 8, vagina; 9, urethra; 10, bladder; 11, vesicouterine recess; 12, fundus of uterus; 13, external iliac vessels; 14, ovarian ligament; 15, uterine tube; 16, suspensory ligament of ovary.

Figure 10.4: 1, fundus; 2, peritoneum (serous layer); 3, oviduct; 4, myometrium; 5, endometrium; 6, anatomical internal os; 7, lateral fornix; 8, external os; 9, vagina; 10, cervix; 11, isthmus; 12, cornu; 13, body.

4 Normal and abnormal sexual development and puberty

a) Turner's syndrome.
b) 45XO.
c) Webbed neck, short stature, wide carrying angle of arms and widely spaced nipples.
d) Low levels of oestradiol with high levels of follicle-stimulating hormone (FSH) and luteinizing hormone (LH).
e) Macroscopically the ovaries appear streaked.
f) There are two phases of treatment. First, at puberty, hormone replacement therapy (HRT) is instigated for the development of secondary sexual characteristics. Second, when the patient wishes to become pregnant, she will require the aid of donor eggs and sperm, which could then be inserted into the uterus.

5 The normal menstrual cycle

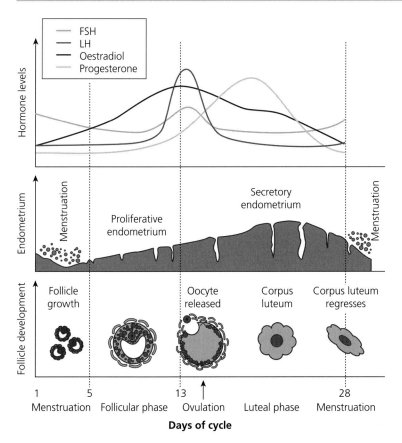

Figure 10.15

6 The normal menstrual cycle

Table 10.5	
Figure 10.6(a)	**Figure 10.6(b)**
Follicular phase	Luteal phase
Proliferative phase	Secretory phase
Glandular and stromal proliferation	Stromal oedema and glandular growth
Pre-ovulation	Post-ovulation
Oestrogen predominates	Progesterone predominates

7 Fertility control

Table 10.6	
Contraceptive method	**Failure rate per 100 women years**
Combined oral contraceptive pill	0.1–1
Progesterone-only pill	1–3
Depo-Provera	0.1–2
Implanon	0
Copper-bearing intrauterine device (IUD)	1–2
Levonorgestrel-releasing IUD	0.5
Male condom	2–5
Female diaphragm	1–15
Persona	6
Natural family planning	2–3
Vasectomy	0.02
Female sterilization	0.13

8 Fertility control

Within the consultation role play ensure the candidate has followed the algorithm as illustrated in Fig. 10.16.

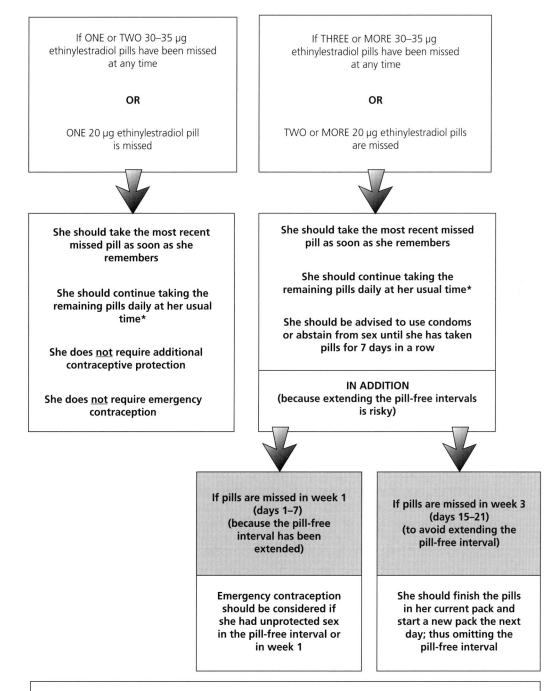

Figure 10.16

9 Fertility control

Table 10.7

Contraceptive method	Inhibition of ovulation	Barrier between gametes	Effect on cervical mucus and prevention of implantation	Toxicity to male gametes
Combined oral contraceptive pill	1*	2†	1	2
Progesterone-only pill	(4%)‡	2	1	2
Depo	1	2	1	2
IUD	2	2	1	1
IUS	2	2	1	2
Condoms	2	1	2	2
Natural family planning	2	1	2	2
Female sterilization	2	1	2	2
Male sterilization	2	1	2	2

*1, Primary mode of action; †2, secondary mode of action; ‡3, only in 4% of women

10 Infertility

a) Polycystic ovary syndrome.

b) Within the consultation role play the candidate should initially counsel the patient regarding the diagnosis and implications of polycystic ovary syndrome. Explain that polycystic ovary syndrome is a condition typified by insulin resistance, an irregular cycle, hirsutism and weight gain. The main problems are anovulation and irregular periods, and women usually present either because of oligomenorrhoea and wanting a regular cycle (these women are usually treated with the combined oral contraceptive pill) or infertility.

One should also explore the long-term implications of unopposed oestrogen as well as the higher risk of endometrial carcinoma later on in life if these patients do not have progesterone. There is also a risk of developing hypercholesterolaemia and non-insulin-dependent diabetes mellitus in later life.

If patients reduce their body mass index by 5 per cent, 30 per cent will achieve ovulation spontaneously and those that do not will be much more receptive to ovulation induction. Ovulation induction can be in the form of oral clomifene citrate or by gonadotrophin therapy if patients are clomifene resistant. It is important to discuss the risks of multiple pregnancy and ovarian hyperstimulation if ovulation induction is embarked upon.

11 Disorders of early pregnancy

a) A threatened miscarriage with a viable intrauterine pregnancy, a non-viable intrauterine pregnancy (silent miscarriage/incomplete miscarriage). Ectopic pregnancy and molar pregnancy cannot be excluded at this time.

b) The diagnosis is a threatened miscarriage with a viable intrauterine pregnancy. Initially, one should reassure the mother that the fetus is viable and the fetal heart can be seen. One should explain the presence of the haematoma has demonstrated some bleeding. It may resolve but she may have further bleeding and may still lose the pregnancy. Initially, one would plan to rescan the pregnancy in 2 weeks' time to confirm viability and see whether the haematoma is resolving. However, you should explain to the patient that she may have further bleeding/pain, which may suggest that she is miscarrying, and if this does occur, she should return to the hospital. She should be given a telephone number to contact the hospital at all times.

c) Explain to the patient that the pregnancy is now not viable and that she will need to have the uterus evacuated. This can be done by expectant, medical or surgical procedures. Surgical evacuation is the most effective, but those managed with expectant and medical management are efficient in 50 per cent and 65 per cent of cases, respectively. One should give the woman contact numbers for support groups and also a contact number if she requires any further information. She should be given advice about subsequent pregnancies and usually one would advise her to refrain from trying to conceive again until she has had a subsequent period.

12 Benign diseases of the uterus and cervix

a) 1, Subserous; 2, submucosal; 3, cervical; 4, intramural; 5, intracavity polyp; 6, pedunculated fibroid.
b) Menorrhagia, pelvic mass, pressure symptoms (urinary frequency), pain (if fibroid is undergoing degeneration).
c) Red, hyaline, cystic, calcification, malignant.

13 Benign diseases of the uterus and cervix

a) The most likely diagnosis is fibroids, but an ovarian cyst with concomitant menorrhagia and adenomyosis is also possible. It is likely that the pelvic mass is causing related pressure symptoms, with urinary frequency resulting from pressure against the bladder and possible right ureteric compression by the fibroid causing renal dilatation.
b) The following investigations would be performed:
   - A full blood count to exclude anaemia, mid-stream urine specimen (MSU) for urinary tract infection (UTI).
   - A pelvic ultrasound scan to determine the nature of the mass to try to distinguish a fibroid from an ovarian mass.
   - A CT scan may be necessary if there are inconclusive results from the ultrasound scan.
   - A renal ultrasound scan/intravenous pyelogram to assess whether there is ureteric obstruction and dilatation of the renal pelvices.
   - Hysteroscopy may be necessary to assess the uterine cavity.
c) As the patient is relatively asymptomatic from her anaemia, she could have iron supplementation rather than risk a blood transfusion. Depending on her fertility wishes, one would need to discuss the following treatments:
   - Mirena, if her uterine cavity is normal; this may give some symptomatic relief but this may be limited to menorrhagia and would not alleviate pressure symptoms.
   - A myomectomy, if the patient wishes to retain fertility.
   - Total abdominal hysterectomy if the patient does not wish to remain fertile.
   - Selective angiographic embolization is a new treatment for fibroids but cannot be used if a woman wants to become pregnant in the future.
   - It is always worth giving adjunctive gonadotrophin-releasing hormone agonist pre-treatment for 2–3 months to reduce the bulk of vascularity of fibroids prior to surgery.

14 Pre-malignant and malignant diseases of the uterus and cervix

a) Colposcopy of the cervix.
b) Acetowhite staining, mosaicism and punctuation.
c) CIN3.

d) Large loop excision of the transformation zone.

e) Human papillomavirus (HPV) strains 16 and 18 are the most commonly associated with cervical cancer.

f) CIN has the potential to develop to an invasive malignancy, although in itself does not have malignant properties. Treatment therefore involves removing the abnormal cells completely down to a depth of 10 mm.

g) Current guidelines recommend a smear and colposcopy at six months after the LLETZ procedure, then a smear by the GP twelve months post-LLETZ and then annually for nine years. After this, if the smears remain normal, the patient can go back to having 3-yearly smears.

15 Infections in gynaecology

a) Fitz-Hugh Curtis syndrome.

b) Chlamydia.

c) Gonorrhoea.

d) The columnar cells of the cervix.

e) Enzyme-linked immunosorbent assay (ELISA). This is the most common investigation; however, it has limited sensitivity. Direct fluorescent antibody (DFA) test can be performed, which is more specific.

f) Doxycycline and azithromycin.

g) Contact tracing and treatment of other sexual partners.

h) Ectopic pregnancy.

16 Infections in gynaecology

a) Kaposi's sarcoma.

b) The condition is the acquired immunodeficiency syndrome (AIDS), which is caused by the human immunodeficiency virus (HIV).

c) 20 per cent of people who acquire HIV have an acute seroconversion illness typified by fever, generalized lymphadenopathy and a maculate erythematous rash, pharyngitis and conjunctivitis. The majority of people are asymptomatic. Affected individuals then develop a steady decline in their immune function over a number of years. This usually presents with non-life-threatening opportunistic infections, such as recurrent candidiasis, shingles and frequent episodes of genital or oral herpes. Hairy oral leukoplakia may come and go, and is pathopneumonic of immunodeficiency. If left untreated, full-blown AIDS will develop usually within 10 years.

d) Transmission is by sexual intercourse and contamination with blood products, such as needle stick injury.

e) It is a single-stranded RNA retrovirus.

f) The gp120 protein binds to the CD4 receptor of the T cells. It then hijacks the cell and uses the viral reverse transcriptase enzyme to produce viral DNA.

g) Seroconversion can be determined by finding antibodies to the gp120 protein. The disease is monitored by measuring the CD4 lymphocyte count.

h) Combination antiviral drugs are used, which target the reverse transcriptase enzyme and viral proteases. These improve life expectancy but are expensive.

17 Urogynaecology

a) 100–150 mL.

b) 10–11.

c) 3.

d) Detrusor overactivity, mixed incontinence or urinary tract infection.

e) Detrusor overactivity /overactive bladder.
f) Previous unsuccessful continence surgery, voiding disorder, neuropathic bladder, investigation prior to embarking on incontinence surgery.

18 Urogynaecology

a) Tension-free vaginal tape (TVT) sling.
b) Urodynamic-proven stress incontinence (USI).
c) Colposuspension.
d) 70–90 per cent long-term success in treating stress incontinence. Long-term risk of poor voiding (5 per cent), *de novo* detrusor overactivity (5 per cent), intermittent self-catheterization (1 per cent) and rectocele.
e) TVT is performed under local anaesthetic, less invasive, shorter hospital stay, quicker recovery, similar success rates but less risk of voiding disorder, *de novo* detrusor overactivity and no increased risk of developing a rectocele.

19 Uterovaginal prolapse

a) 1, internal urethral orifice; 2, vagina; 3, cervix; 4, rectovaginal pouch; 5, rectum; 6, uterosacral ligament; 7, transverse cervical (cardinal) ligament; 8, pubocervical fascia.
b) The mechanisms of support for pelvic organs are:
   • Muscular support; levator ani which forms the pelvic diaphragm.
   • Endofascial supports: uterosacral, cardinal and pubocervical ligaments.
   • The posterior angulation of the vagina, thus preventing pelvic organs falling through the vagina when the patient is standing.

20 Uterovaginal prolapse

a) 1, urethra; 2, bladder; 3, rectum; 4, omentum/small bowel; 5, uterus; 6, vault; 7, urethrocele; 8, cystocele; 9, rectocele; 10, enterocele; 11, uterine prolapse; 12, vault prolapse.
b) Baden–Walker grading:
   • First-degree prolapse is deviation from its anatomical position but not to the level of the hymenal ring/introitus.
   • Second-degree prolapse is deviation of the organ from its anatomical position to the level of the introitus but not beyond.
   • Third-degree prolapse is deviation of the organ from its anatomical position beyond the hymenal ring.

21 The menopause

Within the consultation role play the candidate should explore:

a) Indications and contraindications for HRT. Absolute contraindications include contemporary or suspected pregnancy, suspicion of breast cancer, suspicion of endometrial cancer, acute active liver disease, uncontrolled hypertension or confirmed venous thrombotic event. Relative contraindications include the presence of uterine fibroids, a history of benign breast disease, unconfirmed venous thromboembolic episode, chronic stable liver disease and migraine.
b) Mode of delivery: topical, oral, transdermal and subcutaneous implant.
c) Effects on metabolism: bone (arrests and reverses bone loss), cardiovascular system (reduces vasomotor symptoms, alters lipid profile and increases risk of venous thrombosis), genitourinary system (reduces atrophy) and central nervous system.

d) Progesterone is required to protect the endometrium in women who have not had a hysterectomy.
e) Sequential HRT for women below fifty four or who have been amenorrhoeic for less than two years, and continuous combined HRT for women over fifty four who have been amenorrhoeic for more than two years.

22 Common gynaecological procedures

a) Rigid hysteroscope.
b) Post-menopausal bleeding, irregular menstruation/intermenstrual bleeding in women over the age of 35, persistent menorrhagia, persistent discharge, suspected uterine malformation and suspected Asherman's syndrome.
c) Complications include perforation of the uterus and cervical damage at the time of cervical dilatation, risk of infection and ascending of infection.

23 Common gynaecological procedures

a) This is a laparoscopic view of endometriosis. Endometriosis is scored using the American fertility scoring system.
b) The instrument is called a laparoscope.
c) The indications for laparoscopy include suspected ectopic pregnancy, undiagnosed pelvic pain, tubal patency testing, and sterilization or an operative laparoscopy.
d) Patients need advising about potential complications that include damage to intra-abdominal structures, such as the bowel or major blood vessels. Herniation through port sites is also possible through larger port sites, such as a 10 mm or larger port.

Index

Note: Only items mentioned in questions have been indexed (by page number), with the exception of the short answer questions where the answer appears on the same page as the question.